AS WE GO TO PRESS . . .

On March 30, 1982, the Food and Drug Administration approved the first drug to relieve the symptoms of Herpes. The drug is Acyclovir and is to be marketed by the developers, the Burroughs-Wellcome Company, in the form of an ointment by the trade name of Zovirax. It was reported that the drug will be available for prescription dispensing by pharmacists within thirty days.

As I have spoken of this drug in the book, the publishers wish me to make a further comment even though the main text is in the printing process and cannot be changed at this time.

Acyclovir is a synthetic compound that is thought to work by interrupting DNA production so that the replicating process of the Herpes virus is effectively halted. Dr. Gertrude Elion of Burroughs-Wellcome is reported to have described the process with the statement, "The virus commits suicide."

This mechanism of action is reported to effectively remove a major problem with antiviral drugs in that Acyclovir will destroy the Herpes-infected cell without damaging the normal cells which surround them.

Safety studies in animals have shown no significant adverse effects from the drug. There was no statistical effect upon the unborn young when the animals were given the experimental form of the medication. In short-term tests there were no links to cancer. The drug apparently penetrates the tissues of the brain and may be useful in treatment of that serious problem.

Acyclovir has been tested in an ointment for ophthalmic Herpes, as an intravenous injection for use with immunocompromised and normal patients, as a topical ointment (the only method of administration authorized to date), and as an oral medication.

The drug may shorten the course of an episode of Herpes, but it is not claimed at this time as a cure for the disease. Some of the studies have shown that there is a shortening of the time of virus shedding (the number of days that the virus can be found in the active lesions or in the tissues) but all have not confirmed this result.

It is to be pointed out that the drug does not prevent the transmission of the disease from one part of one's own body to another part or from one individual to another. The same precautions that I have described in detail in the text of the book must still be carried out.

I am encouraged that the Food and Drug Administration has authorized a drug for the treatment of Herpes. I am somewhat surprised by the authorization of the medication in the ointment base, as reports from the Utah College of Medicine, the University of Washington, and other research centers do not share the enthusiasm that the drug manufacturers portray. In my experience, ointments do not reach the source of the virus which may be buried deep in the nerve tissues.

It is my belief that the administration of Acyclovir by the intravenous or the oral route will show more significant results but I shall be watching with great interest the clinical reports on the drug, Zovirax.

The article that I reviewed, which announced the approval of the Food and Drug Administration authorization, appeared in *The Los Angeles Times* of March 31st, 1982. It was written by staff writer Penny Pagano and was as follows: "The FDA's announcement, following an eight-month evaluation of the drug, made the United States the first country to approve a drug product for treatment of genital herpes." This statement is, of course, in complete error as there have been medications for the treatment of genital Herpes authorized in at least fifty-two other nations of the world. Some of these have been used effectively for years and are described in the text of the book.

ADVANCE PRAISE FROM RESPECTED MEDICAL PROFESSIONALS

HERPES:
CAUSE
&
CONTROL

WILLIAM H. WICKETT, JR., M.D.

PINNACLE BOOKS   NEW YORK

HERPES: CAUSE AND CONTROL

Copyright © 1982 by William H. Wickett, Jr., M.D.

An original Pinnacle Books edition, published for the first time anywhere.

First printing, June 1982

ISBN: 0-523-41804-3

Illustrations by Ron Roesch

Printed in the United States of America

PINNACLE BOOKS, INC.
1430 Broadway
New York, New York 10018

14   13   12   11   10   9   8   7   6

DEDICATION

To Wick, my forever partner in all things, without whose encouragement, prodding, ideas, criticism, reading, reading, rereading—and pervasive love —this book would not have been completed.

THIS PUBLICATION IS DESIGNED TO PROVIDE THE AUTHOR'S OPINION OF THE SUBJECT MATTER COVERED. THIS BOOK IS SOLD WITH THE UNDERSTANDING THAT NEITHER THE AUTHOR NOR THE PUBLISHER IS ENGAGED IN RENDERING MEDICAL ADVICE. THE INFORMATION HAS BEEN TAKEN FROM REPORTS THE AUTHOR BELIEVES ACCURATE, BUT NEITHER THE AUTHOR NOR THE PUBLISHER GUARANTEES THE ACCURACY OF SUCH REPORTS. THE AUTHOR AND PUBLISHER SPECIFICALLY DISCLAIM ANY LIABILITY, LOSS OR RISK INCURRED AS A RESULT OF THE USE AND APPLICATION, EITHER DIRECTLY OR INDIRECTLY, OF ANY ADVICE OR INFORMATION PRESENTED IN THIS BOOK.

ACKNOWLEDGMENTS

The author wishes to thank Newport Pharmaceuticals International, Inc. for permission to reprint charts appearing on pages 56, 95, 167, 168; and Ronald Roesch, whose illustrations appear on pages 29, 33, 40, 42, 95.

Contents

Introduction

WHY A BOOK ON
HERPES VIRUS DISEASE?

In the last ten years Herpes virus disease has become epidemic. It has emerged from being considered a nuisance problem of fever blisters to a pestilence of major proportions. Genital Herpes has replaced gonorrhea as the most common sexually transmitted disease. In veneral disease frequency, syphilis is far behind.

Up to 500,000 persons in the United States this year will fall victim, for the first time, to primary genital Herpes. An estimated 10 million to 15 million people will continue to experience the frustrations of secondary recurrences. Researchers at the Center for Disease Control in Atlanta, Georgia, estimate that 30% of the sexually active American population have been exposed. Reports from other nations point to similar statistics in Canada, Japan, and the countries of Europe.

A book on Herpes is needed not only because of the prevalence, but also because of an astonishing lack of knowledge about the disease. That lack applies to physicians as well as patients. When I was in medical school, genital Herpes was not recognized, and it has been only in the last five or six years that much public information has been available on the subject. Few doctors have learned enough about the complexities of Herpes to properly counsel their patients.

This book, although primarily directed toward the intelligent layperson, may also serve as a counseling aid to physicians and other health-related professionals.

My experience as a doctor in private practice, as a physician in Zimbabwe, Africa, and as one who has delivered over 4,000 babies, did not prepare me for the things I found when I left private practice in 1966 to become staff physician and then, three years later, the Director of Medical Services at California State University, Fullerton. College-age persons, those who are working full-time and those who remain in school, are often neglected in their medical care. The 18- to 25-year-old students are usually left out of the mainstream of medical service. They no longer feel comfortable in seeing their pediatrician. They are uneasy in relating inner secrets to their parents' personal physician or to their mother's gynecologist. They are often financially distressed. Many feel abandoned by the medical care system.

At most of the great universities and colleges of our country this problem is being handled by the school itself. Excellent care by physicians of many specialties from psychiatry to dermatology and gynecology, as well as highly trained family practitioners, nurse practitioners, and physical therapists is being furnished. California State University, Fullerton, provides, in addition to the physicians and nurses, full clinical laboratory service, X ray, and pharmacy care. This center is housed in a $2,000,000 building which, with its services and staff, is available to every student.

This was the situation when the epidemic of Herpes began. And it began in the age group of people like our students, the 18- to 25-year-olds who felt they were without medical care.

The inundation of cases of Herpes revealed to me that there is far more need than I had ever imagined. The problem is still growing in scope.

The first realization of the magnitude of the epidemic

2

began to strike me forcibly about the time that we were requested to participate in a major research program relating to Herpes.

The force of that first impression grew daily until I was convinced that a book on Herpes virus disease had to be written.

Credits

My sincere thanks to those friends and supporters who did so much to assist in the writing of this book. Without their help, ideas, hard work, and good sense, this project would have been far more difficult.

To Anne Cross, my daughter, friend, and critic, without whose patient love and editing I would have wallowed in the mire of the language of science and been more bogged in verbosity. We completed the book with Anne still daughter, friend, and critic.

To Bob Settineri, colleague and friend, for the use of his clever brain, his biological expertise, his encouragement and enthusiasm, and his time-consuming work extracting information upon which much of the authority for the book is based.

To Ron Roesch, for his fine sense of art and the ability to simplify the complicated into the understandable.

To Pat Teal and Sandy Watt, my agents, whose idea started this whole project, for interest, enthusiasm, and for coping with my naiveté.

4

To Gaye Tardy, editor, critic, and supporter, and to all the other people of Pinnacle Books, Inc., for their encouragement and work.

To Newport Pharmaceuticals International, Inc., for support and use of materials from their published research projects.

To the members of the Falbag Club, non-medical friends, who read the manuscript with candor and support. I cherish their opinion and their very individual selves.

To the staff of the Health Center, California State University, Fullerton, whose over-and-above teamwork contributed to the research project into Herpes virus disease, and added a caring, compassionate facet to the knowledge of the disease.
  It is with sadness and deep regret that as I was compiling this last section of the book Jean and I learned of the murder, in Thailand, of my friend and former associate, Dr. Helen Morton. Dr. Morton was the first Medical Director of the Health Service, C.S.U.F. She gave her life for the hill people of Thailand. I add my thanks to her, for she taught me much about contagious disease and medical care of young adults. I shall miss her.

Author's Note

The author and publisher disclaim responsibility for any adverse effects or consequences resulting from any treatment, action, or the application of any of the procedures or preparations by any person reading or following the information contained herein.

The publication of this book does not constitute the practice of medicine. No one should commence taking drugs or discontinue a prescribed drug regimen without first consulting a physician or pharmacist.

Foreword

Jane, this book is written for you, even though I don't know you. You came to my lecture at California State University, Fullerton, and left frightened and in tears. I saw you leave and I couldn't get to you to talk further and I still hurt with you.

David, I'm writing for you, too. You exploded into my office and in desperation you called out, "I just gave cancer to my fiancée! What can I do?"

Dr. Joe Robertson, I'm also writing for you. You called me to ask about treatment for your patients and frustratedly sought advice to give them about Herpes.

And this book is written especially for the millions of women and men who have Herpes and who are frightened, in pain, and who may be misinformed.

Jane appeared at a seminar in which I was speaking. She had a special problem and asked a question at the end of the lecture. "What is the relationship between Herpes and pregnancy?"

My colleague and friend, Professor Jack Bradshaw, an authority on the scientific aspect of the disease, related the statistics of the sometimes devastating effects in the infant.

Jane then asked, "What is the treatment?"

I pompously launched into an oration about Caesarean Section surgery for delivery.

My colleague and I left Jane with her questions

poorly answered and her fears intensified. She walked from the lecture in tears for she had Herpes—and she was pregnant. My inadequate attempt to answer her questions had only reinforced her concerns. Jane wants a perfect baby and she wants to deliver her infant by natural childbirth. If Jane has active Herpes lesions at the time of delivery, normal programs are probably not advisable.

David's dramatic entrance into my office not only caught my attention but also necessitated lengthy discussion to moderate his fears. He had had sex with his fiancée the night before. The day he pushed past my secretary, he had read an article from which he concluded that Herpes causes cancer of the cervix. His hasty interpretation of the information had caused emotional anguish for the girl he loved as well as for him. And a late dinner for me.

Dr. Robertson's question is one that I hear often, "What can I do and say about Herpes?" We in Medicine don't know all the answers yet but we are gaining information. The disease has some enormous emotional factors that need explanation and wise and patient counsel.

Who ever you may be, this book is also written for you as personally as I can make it: to share my experiences in the investigation of Herpes; to describe what is known about the disease and how one contracts it; to refer to the treatments available; and to discuss hopes for future control.

At California State University, Fullerton, in 1976, we were asked to undertake a research study to test a new drug and its effectiveness against Herpes virus disease. We knew that the ailment is found more often in college-age persons, so we decided on a study series involving a large group, 100 cases proven to have the malady by culture of the Herpes simplex hominus virus, the cause of the problem.

8

The research used what is called a double-blind technique: fifty patients were given the experimental drug which we were testing and fifty other patients were given a placebo. A placebo is a dummy pill which has no effect on the body but which appears similar in every way to the active medication. All patients were volunteers and all procedures were explained to them in detail.

In order to promote impartial reporting of results, a double-blind study utilizes a certified procedure organization which keeps secret the code that lists which patient receives which substance, the active one or the placebo. Only after the study is completed and all data are filed with the certifying agency, is the code made available to the researcher. At that time we were able to correlate the results with the treatment. We could then determine whether or not those patients receiving the active medication were the ones who improved.

Neither I, nor the doctors, nurses, technologists, and pharmacists working with me, nor the patients themselves, knew who was receiving the drug and who was given the placebo. Because of these requirements we had to make very critical observations on the effect of the disease upon each patient. I personally examined each one and we made extensive physical, virological, clinical, and laboratory determinations. I serially photographed the lesions of each patient as he or she progressed. We collected information about who had Herpes, how it may have been contracted, about pain and other symptoms, about the age of the patients, about any other medicines the patient was taking (birth control pills, antibiotics, etc.), and whether this current episode was a recurrence or an initial attack of the disease.

The results of the accumulated data were astonishing.

Our first surprise was the number of people who answered the small want ads we placed in the local papers. We announced that we were interested in doing something about Herpes and asked for volunteers. People came in droves! They came by themselves. They were referred by the Health Department. They came from hospitals, from Free Clinics, and from private physicians. Our one hundred patients were obtained in one half the time we had estimated.

Secondly, we were confounded by the universal sense of fright, frustration, and false information among the many who volunteered.

The third surprising result was found in the laboratory by my colleague, Dr. Jack Bradshaw, Professor of Molecular Biology. He determined that most of the patients who had Herpes also had a lowered resistance factor to virus disease. This means that the ability of the body to combat disease was significantly less in Herpes patients than in persons without the condition.

I am convinced there is hope for control of this disease. That's what this book is all about. It is for you, Jane, and for you, David. It's also for you, Dr. Robertson, as you struggle with the problems of Herpes simplex in the everyday practice of medicine. I believe that if each of you has more information about Herpes, your emotions will be more stable, and your reactions more logical. I hope that the information contained herein will ease the fear misinformation breeds, and will reflect the hope of the new approaches to this epidemic problem.

Chapter 1

WHY ME?

So the doctor said, "You've got Herpes————."

And you said, "Oh, my God!"

And he said so easily, "Just forget it! It will go away. Just don't do anything that will make it worse. Take some aspirin for the pain. And be especially careful not to worry."

"How did I get it?"

"Don't you know? You're the one that's got it. If it gets more sore, call me and we'll think about a consultation."

He washed his hands—twice—and then showed you to the office door, seeming to take care not to touch you. You're stunned! You think, I've got Herpes! What a shocker!

Why is he so cool all of a sudden? Is he thinking, "You've got V.D.!"

You furtively return to the waiting room. All the patients look up—and somehow seem to know. The outer door appears to be a football field away.

When you get home you go straight to your room. You feel worse than when you went to the doctor. Your head is in a whirl and the sores that took you there hurt like crazy. Your lymph glands are sore—the ones you didn't know were swollen until he pointed them out.

11

Your head aches and you cannot seem to get away from it. Your eyes are tired and burn.

Yes, you do have Herpes. The doctor's diagnosis was correct, but his helpfulness was lousy. You have it—so what do you do about it?

One of your first questions probably is, "Why me?" And that's difficult to answer. But it's what I want to tell you about. It is not to sit in judgment of you. Or to tell you to forget it. But it is to try to explain to you the essentials I have observed about the disease, the reasons why it acts as it does, and some of the hopes for the future.

You are still asking, "Why me? Why did I get it? Why didn't some of my friends get it when we did the same things?"

It is impossible to complete the explanation to those questions in one quick sentence, for Herpes is a very complicated problem. Basically, a person contracts Herpes in one of two ways: exposure to a high degree of infectious material, or lowered resistance to the agent that causes the disease, the Herpes virus.

EXPOSURE TO INFECTIOUS MATERIAL

The sores of many diseases weep a serum that contains a large amount of the agent that causes that specific disease.

Herpes is caused likewise by a specific virus that is like no other. (Viruses are unique and will be discussed in Chapter 3.)

The virus of Herpes can enter the body through any defect in the skin or mucous membrane. These structures have a defensive function like that of plastic wrap that fits tightly and completely over the bowl of Jell-O salad which remained after yesterday's dinner. The plastic helps to repel any contaminant that might get into the food. Should there be a hole in the plastic,

12

molds, fungi, bacteria—or viruses—could sneak into the gelatin and cause it to spoil.

When there is a defect, such as a cut or a scratch in the skin or mucous membrane of the body, this same course of events can happen. In this book we are mainly discussing viruses—and one in particular. When there is a flaw in the protective covering of the body Herpes simplex hominis virus can enter!

LOWERED RESISTANCE

Another way of contracting Herpes is through lowered resistance. When our immune defense is down, there is a greater possibility of an infection taking hold and beginning to cause symptoms.

The immune defenses of the body are the biochemical barriers that protect us from disease. To illustrate the immune defense system we might picture a lake filled with sparkling water. Fresh streams bring a new supply of nutrient continuously so that life below the surface can be vigorous and healthy. The streams keep the lake full. At the lower end of the lake the water spills into the river that flows down the mountain. Any waste is expelled downstream. This lovely cycle of nature maintains the beauty and the purity of the ecosystem.

However, sometimes there is no rain; the streams become rivulets and then dry up completely. The run-off stops and the water from the lake evaporates. No waste is discharged. The water level falls, and all sorts of problems begin to show up. Old tree snags catch boat bottoms and fish lines. Rocks begin to appear that are hazards to navigation and swimming. The acidity of the water changes ever so slightly. The oxygen content decreases and life is in jeopardy.

Our human system is like that. When the level of resistance has deteriorated all sorts of hazards become apparent. Within each of us are viruses lurking dormant in various parts of our bodies. This is particularly true of the Herpes virus which seems to be asleep in nerve tissues. Our immune abilities keep the virus quiet in times when there is nothing to lower those defenses. However, like the drought times affect the lake, something may suppress those immune activities. When this happens we no longer have the ability to fight off disease—the water level of the lake has fallen so that no waste is discharged. Upon still further depression of our defenses, the virus begins to stir and respond to the change within our bodies—the tree snags and rocks begin to appear. This phenomenon accentuates the process so that any weakened area of our body is liable to be attacked by the virus. The sores begin to show up where there is a place of weakness. And—like the lake that becomes polluted—we have an episode of Herpes.

In the opening dialogue, I wrote about how you may have felt when you were first told of having Herpes. You were depressed by such news. Justifiably so, for this disease is one that we really don't know much about, and so far there is no approved treatment. In my homely illustration, the doctor's manner was atrocious. I don't know many physicians who will treat a patient like that, failing to explain what is happening, and further, being extremely judgmental. But I do know some. Unfortunately, this sequence of events occurs all too frequently when the diagnosis is that of Herpes. Many physicians are confused by the disease and don't know what advice to give.

Questions about Herpes occur not only to you but also to me. One of my own is why, when I have spent seven years working intimately with persons so afflicted, have I never had an outbreak of the disease. Neither have the nurses who worked with me, nor the laboratory technologists who handled the highly con-

14

taminated specimens which we collected from patients having the problem.

As I said before, Herpes is a complicated disease. In Chapter 2 we will begin to try to explain some of the things we do know about it by describing symptoms and signs and discussing the different types of the disease's manifestations. Actual examples of cases I have treated and cared for personally will be presented.

All the names used in this book that relate to patients or case histories are fictional. Certain aspects of the cases have been altered to protect the personal, sacred, and inviable relationship of confidence that exists between a doctor and her or his patients. The data which is described have been published widely in national and international medical and microbiological science journals and are not confidential. The opinions expressed are my own and I do not speak for anyone else relative to treatments and findings. In this work I am not promoting or criticizing any course of treatment which others may advocate, but I am relating what my own experience and research have found.

Chapter 2

WHAT IS HERPES?

Herpes is caused by a virus. The official name of the condition is Herpes simplex virus disease. Often, it is also called HSV, but for this work I shall use the term "Herpes" whenever the condition is mentioned. The term is a Greek word meaning to "creep," but with the connotation of creeping like a serpent. This seems to be an accurate description.

Historically, the symptoms have been noted since ancient times and were probably confused with other skin conditions such as syphilis, eczema, Herpes zoster (shingles), and even leprosy. The disease was named in 1736 by a French physician, Jean Astruc, who described the condition quite accurately. Unfortunately his research work was lost for 200 years and has only recently been rediscovered. But two centuries of progress in treating the disease was forfeited.

The Herpes simplex virus was not isolated until recently, and it wasn't until the 1960s that the two strains of the virus were identified. Some clever person named these strains Type 1 and Type 2.

Herpes is an epidemic problem in the United States, Canada, Europe, and Japan. It is a disease which is affected greatly by anxiety and stress. As these traits are often considered to be characteristic of the developed nations, it may be that many countries of Asia, South

America, and Africa are not as aware of the problems as we. Race, however, has little to do with the incidence of the condition. Some of the patients in our clinic were black, some were Hispanic, but they were predominantly white, as is the population of the area.

In 1968 a major report inferred that Herpes Type 1 causes lesions (sores) above the waist and Herpes Type 2 causes lesions below the waist. This is basically true. However, because of our changing sexual mores and an increase in oral-genital sex, the virus may get mixed up. Sometimes we find a reversal in the site of the infection: Type 1 virus may be found in the genital lesions and Type 2 may be the cause of oral lesions or even sores of the eyes.

This chapter will deal with the symptoms of the disease, a description of the blisters, where they are located, and how the disease progresses. There are some differences in the effects in women and men. I shall describe those variations and also the results of infections with Type 1 and Type 2 virus. The dissimilarities between infections of the lips (Herpes labialis) and Herpes of the genital organs (Herpes genitalis) will be outlined.

(Please see Figure C at the end of this chapter for additional help in understanding the locations of the lesions.)

FEVER BLISTERS

Fever blisters or cold sores are the most common evidence of Herpes. They appear annually on the lips of approximately 30,000,000 people. The sores begin twelve to thirty-six hours after exposure to the sun or kissing someone who has a fever blister. The blisters are usually located on the lower lip, though in some cases the upper or even both lips may be involved.

The first symptom a patient seems to notice is a vague burning of the skin and often I am told, "I guess

I bit my lip." Soon redness and swelling occur. Occasionally the lips balloon to almost twice the normal size.

A blister is the next event to be noted. This may be at the same time as the swelling or it may precede it by a day or two. The blister is often one to four centimeters in length (one fourth to one inch) and the full width of the lip. Because of the softness of the lip tissue the blister will rupture easily. There is often a little bleeding that results. The pain at this time is quite annoying. This stage of the development of the condition lasts about one day.

Gradually a crust forms over the area where the blister has been. The crust is often dark red or blackish. It cracks easily and causes pain and frequently enough bleeding to cause a person to dab at the lip with a handkerchief or a tissue. In about a week, the crust disappears and only a little inflammation (redness) remains. This fades slowly over the next few days.

Cold sores are seen far more frequently in the summer. It is my opinion that the ultraviolet light which occurs in higher density in the sunshine of those months may be the "trigger" that sets off the chain of events which ends in the typical blisters.

During the summer the orbit of the earth brings us much closer to the sun. Consequently, the ultraviolet radiation is much increased. That is one reason why we tan in the summer more than we do in the winter. The winter sun is farther from the earth and the ultraviolet rays are less concentrated.

The bleb on the lip often is the response in the body when some trigger sets off the episode. Frequently patients relate that they have the sore in the same place time after time.

Fever blisters also occur, as the name implies, following fever. Any infection within the body that causes a generalized elevation of body temperature may have, as one of its manifestations, a fever blister.

19

Incidentally, the term "trigger" is one I have used several times already. I will use it many times in this book. The word may be a Bill Wickettism which science seems to have picked up—or maybe it's vice versa. However, in the context of this book the term refers to an event, a substance, a virus or biological irritant, or even a stress that seems to set off or start a Herpes episode.

Ted was a student at our university. He loved to water ski and every possible weekend he would leave Fullerton on a Friday evening, make the six-hour drive to the Colorado River, and sack out. Up early, Ted would ski in the brilliant desert sunshine all day Saturday and Sunday and get thoroughly sunburned in the process. He would return home Sunday night. Every other weekend he carried out this activity—exposing himself to about twenty hours of ultraviolet irradiation. By Monday morning following his return, he would develop a blazing blister on the right side of his lower lip. The lesion never occurred on the left side and never on the upper lip.

I talked to Ted at length of the hazards of repeated exposure to the sun, but he decided that water skiing was one of his joys and was worth the discomfort of the inflammation. The fire in his lip and the enlarged lymph glands in his neck that usually accompanied the infection lasted about nine days or until he was ready for the next trek.

I shall speak of Ted several times in future chapters.

CANKER SORES

These nasty little lesions are a puzzle. But they are a part of the many different facets of Herpes.

The mouth is a particularly dirty place. Some of the

20

messiest wounds we doctors treat are human bites. By medical definition these injuries may not be actual bites but occur whenever someone's skin is accidentally or purposely cut on the teeth of another person. A whole cadre of bacteria and viruses can invade the body through the resulting abrasion or laceration. It is nearly impossible to separate the Herpes virus from the many other germs in the mouth and to determine which is the actual cause of the infection.

To further complicate the situation, the cells of the different tissues respond differently to varieties of invaders. There are three separate types of cells in the area of the lips. The cells which comprise the skin are flat and pointed at each end. This type of cell covers the vast majority of the body and, in the area of the mouth extends to the margin of the lips. The lips themselves are a softer and more delicate combination of cells than the skin. The lining tissue of the mouth is composed of still another entirely different type of cells. These are cuboid and under the microscope look like a pile of cardboard cartons stored systematically upon one another.

A particular virus does not usually attack cells of different anatomic characteristics. However, if the exposure is great enough such an event may happen.

Canker sores are small, extremely painful ulcers of the buccal mucosa (the scientific name for the layer of cardboard carton-like cells). Often cankers appear after some trauma. A blow to the face which causes laceration or contusion to the tissues of the mouth may result in the lesions. Even biting one's own cheek not only hurts like sin but also leaves behind the residual of the sores. Certain toxins may be the trigger that starts the problems: walnuts and macadamia nuts are particularly villainous culprits in my family. The reason for this will be discussed in the chapter on Triggers.

21

KERATITIS

One of the serious complications of Herpes Type I is an infection called keratitis. The condition involves the eye. Painful red eyes following fever blisters or genital Herpes require immediate consultation with an ophthalmologist, a physician with experience in treatment of diseases of the eye.

The serious nature of this problem is manifest when one realizes that the tiny ulcers which occur on the cornea or outer surface of the pupil can cause permanent damage. Small scars can be the result. The defect, like a scratch on the lens of a camera, will cause the image which is reflected on the retina of the inner portion of the eye (as on the photographic film) to be diffuse or fuzzy.

Debbie came into our clinic in pain and ill. She had serious Herpetic lesions in the vaginal region and around her mouth. Another problem was that of painful red eyes. The blood vessels were inflamed and light caused her pain. Staining with flourescein (an agent in eye drops that outlines tiny irregularities of the surface of the eye) showed some small ulcers of the cornea. For this problem of keratitis Debbie was referred immediately to an eye clinic to assist in the care of a difficult problem.

HERPES OF THE SKIN

Herpes lesions are not limited to the lips, the eyes, or the genitalia. Occasionally one finds the sores in remote parts of the body.

Walter was an above average student who suffered from a habit not uncommon in persons who are concentrating. He often sucked, chewed, or at least touched to his lips the second joint of the index finger of his left hand.

When he presented himself at the clinic, his main complaint was that of an ulcer at the second joint of the left index finger. Walter had previously seen other physicians who had tested the fester for syphilis, but the local microscopic examination called the dark-field had been negative. In this examination a skilled technician can identify the spirochetes which cause the disease. The blood test for syphilis was also negative.

Walter did have a fever blister and on close questioning, the relationship of putting that particular area of his finger to his lips revealed the answer to the diagnostic puzzle. We became suspicious of Herpes. Both sores, the finger and the lip, revealed positive cultures of Herpes simplex virus, Type 1. This kind of lesion is seen often enough to have been given its own name. It is called a Herpetic Whitlow.

Walter's case illustrates two things about Herpes: one, that Herpes can attack the tough skin covering of the body as well as the softer and more vulnerable mucous membranes; and two, that the condition can spread by direct contact or "autoinoculation."

Josie is a pleasant, genteel lady of 72 years. She came to us as a result of the ads in the newspaper and was by far the oldest person whom I have seen who has been proven to have Herpes simplex virus disease.

Josie related having a single recurrent lesion about the size of a silver dollar on the upper part of her right buttock. The significant fact about her history is that the blister had been recurring about every month for forty years. We were able to culture the virus from the fluid of the infected site.

In addition to this evidence that she did have Herpes, we found another positive test which confirmed the diagnosis. Large cells which have multiple nuclei were found. These giant cells have an odd but quite consistant appearance under the microscope. They are seen in the serum (fluid) which exudes from the sores. Finding these large cells was previously the primary method of making the diagnosis and still is one way of helping to confirm it.

Josie seems to be one of those people whose immune level remains low.

HERPES GENITALIS

Lesions of the genital region can be caused by either Type 2 or Type 1 Herpes simplex virus. The strain of the virus most dominant is Type 2. The sores begin two to twelve days after exposure to someone who has active lesions.

A number of symptoms are common to the disease in both sexes. I shall describe those first and then discuss the particular problems of women. Finally I shall take up the disease as it relates to men, and then to homosexuals.

Symptoms which are seen in both male and female herpetic involvement include enlargement of the lymph glands, fever, and headache. The lymphatic system is one of our vital defenses. Whenever the human body is invaded by an extrinsic substance like a toxin or a virus, the system carries the offender to a place where there is an excellent blood supply. Lymph nodes are such sites and are located in many places throughout the body.

Because of the plentiful blood supply in the nodes, the protective elements of the system can defend against the invaders. It is like some old Western movie scouts leading the band of black-hatted villains into an ambush where there are many good white-hatted cowboys

24

who can do battle—and win! However, during the skirmish there are losses on both sides.

This scenario holds when the body's defenses do battle with the Herpes virus. During the fight, good blood cells are destroyed by the invaders. If our defenses are strong, more of the attackers are eliminated than the cells of our bloodstream, and our system improves until we are cured. However, if our system is weakened, the invaders will destroy the defensive cells and we become more ill.

The lymph glands are usually not palpable (they cannot ordinarily be felt) but during the conflict with the disease elements these glands have the task of localizing the attack and cleaning up any debris left from the battling of the cells. In this event the glands can easily be detected by pressing the fingers gently against the area where they are located. We have all felt such enlarged glands while feeling the area of our neck below the ear when we have had a sore throat. In addition, there are many other clusters of nodes: under the jaw, at the nape of the neck, behind the ears, in the axillae (the arm pits), and in the groin. Many other nodes are not palpable and are located along the course of the intestine and other inaccessible places.

The lymph glands swell in the area close to the site of the infection: in the neck area in cases of severe fever blisters, and in the groin in the cases of genital Herpes. There may be several groups of glands that are enlarged. When the glands are swollen, there is a mild pain or soreness that accompanies pressure on the area. Many patients will not notice the sensitivity until the glands are touched. The swelling lasts during the entire period of the active infection and may remain for some time afterward.

Fever is another common symptom. A temperature elevation of 99.8° to 100.5° is not uncommon. Higher temperatures are not usual unless the patient has a con-

25

current bacterial infection. The fever ordinarily lasts during the first five or six days of the attack and then returns to normal.

Headache is a constant problem that lasts during most of the episode. The discomfort is often in the front portion of the head but seems difficult to define. It is persistent. Sleep makes little difference; a patient will complain of the headache on going to bed and on arising. It is not severe and can usually be controlled by aspirin every 4 to 6 hours.

HERPES LESIONS IN WOMEN

The first symptoms to appear in the genital type of Herpes in women are the usual ones of headache, enlarged lymph nodes, and a mild fever. Sores in the mouth may or may not be present. Burning on urination is common. These symptoms all may appear before the sensitivity begins in the genital area.

The ulcers of the disease may be multiple or there may be just a few. A finding of only one sore is not unusual. The lesions may be distributed widely over the perineum and the vulva, from the mons veneris (in front, where the hair is), over the clitoris, the labia, and the forchet (the area between the posterior portion of the vagina and the anus). Sores may be noted to each side toward the thighs. Lesions in the area of the anus are not uncommon.

The typical lesions of Herpes in women are about one centimeter or one fourth of an inch in diameter and are extremely painful to the touch. The pain is particularly severe in sores which are located on the labia (the lips of the vagina) or the clitoris (the structure that is in front of the vagina and is highly supplied with nerves).

When the labia are involved with the disease process, they may swell to twice the normal size. Clothes or sanitary napkins are an agony. Stylish skintight jeans are a particular problem. I recommend to my patients that they wear loose-fitting cotton shorts or even long dresses with no panties at all.

Sex causes pain when there are lesions. For that reason alone (and there are several others that I will discuss in following chapters) sex should be avoided when anyone has active sores.

It is extremely important to remember that the ulcers of Herpes are also found in the vagina and on the cervix. Outbreak of lesions in those areas are particularly difficult to detect. The inside of the vagina has few nerve endings and the cervix even fewer. Because of this lack of sensation, the lesions are often painless and many women do not sense that there is any problem. Unfortunately, some physicians do not diligently search those areas for visible signs of Herpes if the patient does not complain of pain.

Pain outside of the vagina may be the first sign of a problem. It frequently occurs in the vulvar area. The pain is followed in a matter of hours or days by inflammation which in turn is followed by a blister.

In women the blister phase is often not seen because the vesicle or bleb that contains the fluid is so soft that it ruptures easily. When this happens an ulcer remains. These little holes are sometimes one eighth of an inch deep and have a moist, red, and exquisitely tender surface. The redness changes over the course of a few days to a deep maroon or even a blackish color. During this same time the lesions change from moist to dry.

As stated, there may be few nerve endings inside the vagina so that any ulcers which exist there may not cause pain. However, those ulcers do cause a very irritating fluid to be discharged. The fluid seeps out of the vagina and onto the sensitive surfaces of the vulva and the skin. Itching and soreness frequently result. In addition, because it contains active Herpes virus, the fluid

27

may eventually cause the typical lesions in the vulvar area by autoinoculation.

Velma is a typical example of women who have Herpes. She told me of having sore spots on the vulva. These had been present for three days and were on the right side of the right labia major and near the forchet. On examination two small ulcers one fourth of an inch in diameter were noted. Each was surrounded by a small crater wall and inflammation, and each was covered by a moist exudate. Velma stated that she was taking birth control pills. Other past history of medical problems revealed only that of a urinary tract infection which had been treated successfully.

Velma's course was not out of the ordinary and all lesions had cleared by the time she had been seen in our clinic for eight days.

Marilyn, another typical case, was seen in the clinic three days after symptoms first began. "Sore spots and little cuts on the labia" was the concern that brought her to seek help. She stated that she had not ever had such a problem before. In addition, Marilyn related that she had a burning sensation whenever she urinated. Her last menstrual period occurred a few days before the pain began. Birth control pills were part of her routine.

When I examined Marilyn I found the right labia to be swollen and red. There was moisture in the area and there were three painful red ulcers at the base of the labia near the hymenal ring (the residual tissue of the hymen). Another ulcer was adjacent to the urethra, the small opening through which urine flows out of the body. This structure is near the front of the vagina.

There were also canker sores in Marilyn's mouth.

During the time of observation, Marilyn had no fever and there was no swelling of the lymph nodes. The redness and pain gradually disappeared. Burning on urination lessened and disappeared in three days. By the tenth day after her entry into the clinic no residual of the lesions nor of the canker sores was noted.

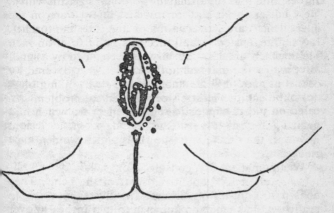

The above drawing illustrates the typical lesions that are noted on the vulva.

HERPES SYMPTOMS IN MEN

In men the genital lesions of Herpes are more localized than those of women. Probably this phenomenon has to do with the anatomy of the area: the penis and scrotum are essentially dry areas but the vulva and vagina are moist. Moisture seems to soften the tissues and causes the surfaces of the skin to break down. The spread of the virus in the serous discharge is wider in women and there is more chance of autoinoculation.

Male patients state that the first symptom of Herpes is often a burning sensation felt in a localized area. The site of the burning feeling may be anywhere in the genital region but is usually on the shaft of the penis or near the corona (the flare at the end of that organ). Burning may be noted on the scrotum.

One or two days after the pain begins, the area becomes inflamed. The redness at first is generalized in the painful site but then it becomes more localized. Next blisters begin to form. At first there are small vesicles which are covered by a tan plastic-appearing layer. The blisters may grow and unite to form large blebs which are like the blisters seen in the course of any first or second degree burn. The vesiculation process continues until about the fourth day of the disease.

At the end of the first week the blisters begin to rupture and ulcers similar to those seen in women are revealed. There is less exudate seeping from the lesions, however, than there is in the sores which women experience.

When a patient first consults a physician, typical blisters are often seen about midshaft of the penis. These consist of a cluster of vesicles. The cluster may be generally oval in shape and one inch to two inches in overall length. The watery blisters may measure one eighth of an inch in height.

When these blisters break, a fluid which is highly contaminated with the Herpes simplex virus seeps out. The discharge may cause satellite vesicles by autoinoculation. The sores are painful to the touch. It is difficult to evaluate but I have the impression that the lesions of women are larger and more painful than those of men.

Sexual stimulation and penile erection cause a bout of pain similar to that caused during the swelling of the clitoris and labia in women. All of the structures are very tender, and sexual arousal and activity accentuate the problem.

The ulcers dry up during the next period of days. The inflammation which surrounds the lesions ebbs and finally a crust forms; it is brownish or slightly red and is formed by the secretions of the sore together with a few blood cells. The layer is hard and, at first, firmly adherent to the underlying ulcer.

In six or seven days the crusts begin to fall off. This process is nearly completed in forty-eight hours. There may be a small amount of bleeding when the crusts separate. Left behind is a patch of inflammation roughly identical in size and shape to the area of vesiculation. In an indefinite number of days the redness fades and the lesions disappear.

Lymph node enlargement follows the same course in men and women and usually is completed with the fading of the inflammation.

Herpes in men reminds me of a first or second degree burn caused by a hot stove. In a few hours after touching the stove a large blister forms. When the blister breaks (and it may be tough and slower to break than a blister of Herpes), there is an area of ulceration revealed. This area is very tender. If the burn has destroyed the deep layer of the skin, primary healing cannot occur. The growing, regenerating cells of the skin are missing and healing is slower. Scarring results.

A similar situation occurs when the Herpes lesions penetrate deeper tissues; a scar is the result. Scarring is not usual but is sometimes seen on the shaft of the penis where the skin is thin and very tender. Subsequent episodes may recur in the same site causing the skin to become parchment-like and shiny.

Occasionally, the blisters are merely pencil-point-size ulcers. This type of lesion seems to be less painful and to heal more rapidly.

Steve had a rash on his penis which had been present for five days before he came to the clinic. He stated that there were few new lesions and that some of the older ones had started to dry up. A few of the sores still had some moisture. He said there was also a sore on the

31

scrotum. Steve denied ever having had this type of problem before.

When I examined Steve and questioned him he told of painful and frequent urination and painful sexual intercourse. He admitted to not being hungry and even stated that he was slightly nauseated.

Physical examination revealed large lymph nodes in the groin, and swelling in the area of three ulcers on the dorsum of the penis, the top front portion.

During the time we cared for Steve a few new vesicles formed. One of these blisters was still present ten days after we first saw him. The painful urination was no longer present after the second day of our study of Steve.

Peter reported to me that he had Herpes intermittently for seven years. At first the lesions were only on his lips but eventually the sores began to be evident on the penis. When first seen in the clinic, Pete complained of a sore in the left corner of his mouth and an ulcer on the inside of the urethral opening of the penis. He told of having had twenty to thirty episodes of Herpes since it began seven years ago.

Peter's physical examination revealed enlarged lymph glands in his neck and in the groin. There was a typical ulcer of Herpes near the opening of the urethra. The lymph node enlargement persisted during the study.

The following sketch illustrates the typical site of Herpes lesions in men.

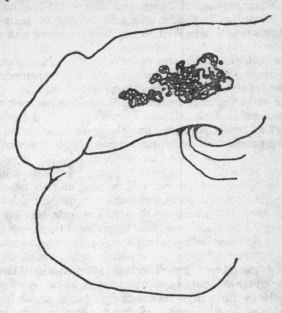

HERPES GLADIATORUM

The grand name of this type of Herpes is applied to those who contract the disease as a result of athletic contests. It is listed in the male section only because fewer women participate in contact sports. The most frequent athletes that experience this problem are wrestlers.

When two athletes are engaged in all-out combat on a mat where many others have also dropped their sweat and virus particles, the virus can get into the skin surface. A mat burn, a scratch, or a minor laceration can become a major Herpes problem. Herpes virus Type 1 is the usual cause.

Atlas was a wrestler. Not a heavyweight he, but a smaller variety. Agile and quick, he could often pin his opponent with sudden moves in which he would dive to the canvas and catch the less active competitor off guard. He was one of the champions of the university team and seemed to be headed for the National Championships.

When I saw Atlas he was far from holding up the world or even his part of the team. Apparently, when diving to gain a hold on his opponent, he had abraded his left shoulder on the wrestling mat. A few days later typical lesions of Herpes had begun, and though the trainer had sprayed the area with anesthetic and cortisone, the lesions progressed. I had to rule him out of further competition until the lesions were much less of a hazard to those with whom he was competing.

My experience has not yet encountered Herpes among that exhibition sport that seems to be growing in popularity, "female mud-wrestling." But it seems likely that, in such an environment, it could well happen.

HERPES LESIONS IN HOMOSEXUALS

The location and distribution of the sores of Herpes vary to a degree depending on the mode of sexual activity experienced by the individual.

When Pamela came to the clinic she had a serious infection of Herpes. Lesions covered the mons, the clitoris, the labia and the forchet. There were probably more than sixty individual sores. She was in agony. No ulcers were found inside the vagina or on the cervix.

Pam's story revealed oral-genital sexual contact with Dorothy three days before. Pam described Dorothy's fever blister to be on her lower lip.

Pam brought her friend to the clinic the next day. Examination proved that both Pam and Dorothy had lesions from which we cultured Type 1 virus.

Matt was found to have lesions of the anus. These were moist, as is that part of the anatomy. The lesions in that particular area progress in a similar manner in both males and females because moisture is the dominant physiological factor.

Upon questioning, we found we were already treating Matt's sexual partner, Tim, for blisters located on the shaft of the penis. Tim had apparently contracted Herpes from a sexual contact with a woman who was not part of our study.

FLARE-UPS OR RECURRENCES

Herpes episodes vary greatly in duration, severity, and frequency. Some attacks last a few days, but others seem to be almost continuous. Some cause severe pain, others very little.

The initial episode of Herpes is usually the most severe and the longest lasting. Often that bout lasts ten to twelve days.

The episodic nature of the disease is such that recurrences are frequent. They do not always recur in a definite time pattern, but the majority of patients report that their bouts recur approximately every six weeks. Recurrences ordinarily decrease in severity and frequency.

Although our research study did not collect data relative to the question, it seems to me that six episodes is about the average total number before cessation of recurrences. The term I use here is the "average" number

35

of recurrences—not the "normal" number. Some patients have only one occurrence. That seems to be enough to boost their immunity level so that there are no more. Other patients have fifteen to twenty before the battle of the body with the virus is finally won. A very few people continue to have bouts for years with no apparent build-up of immunity. Josie, the senior lady whom I previously mentioned, is in this latter group.

HERPES ENCEPHALITIS

Herpes simplex virus encephalitis (Herpes of the brain) is probably a rare condition. At least the confirmation of the diagnosis is rare. It is difficult to prove except by means of virus cultures from brain tissue. In the cases confirmed to date it is a devastating problem.

It is speculated that the frequency of its occurrence is increasing but, as with other types of Herpes infections, no one is really sure. It has been estimated that 4.000 cases may occur in the United States each year. This is fewer than the number for encephalitis caused by the mumps virus or the insect-borne viruses, but the mortality and the residual effects cause it to rank as a very serious problem.

HERPES IN INFANTS

The usual cause of Herpes infection in infants is the Type 2 virus, which is contacted by the newborn as he or she passes through the vagina during the birth process. When genital Herpes lesions are present in the mother at the time of vaginal delivery, it has been estimated that forty to sixty percent of the infants will be infected with the disease. About one half of these infants will suffer serious brain damage or even die from Herpes encephalitis. This incidence of tragic problems

36

is greatly reduced when delivery by Caesarean section is performed before there is a rupture of the membranes (the water breaks).

In relatively rare instances, Herpes is acquired by the newborn from other sources than the mother. The result of this type of spread to a baby causes the same devastating effect, however. Separating the newborn infant from persons with active lesions caused by Herpes Type 1 or Type 2 is absolutely imperative. Parents, friends, and brothers or sisters with fever blisters or other Herpes sores must NOT be allowed to kiss or fondle the newborn in ANY circumstances. This rule even applies to grandmothers and aunts!

It is extremely important for women who have had Herpes at any time in the past to report this history to their obstetricians. It is also just as necessary for the one in charge of the obstetrical care to inquire about the patient's history of Herpes and to search diligently for the lesions. The examination should concentrate not only on the skin of the mother, but also on the inside of the vagina and the surface of the cervix.

As the pregnancy approaches term, caution should be exercised. One of the problems with Herpes during pregnancy is that of prematurity. About fifty percent of such pregnancies terminate between the thirtieth to the thirty-fifth week. The normal length of gestation in women is forty weeks. Monitoring of the signs of Herpes during the last weeks of the pregnancy is an essential part of the care, and if active Herpes is found, delivery by Caesarean section is probably advised.

HERPES ENCEPHALITIS IN ADULTS AND CHILDREN

Encephalitis in persons older than infants is a very difficult diagnosis to make with certainty. The only definitive method is by brain biopsy, which necessitates a surgical procedure taken during a time of risk. So it leaves us as doctors in the insecure position of treating a patient for a very serious problem with only our clinical opinion to rely upon.

The statistics state that the mortality rate of Herpes encephalitis is high, but this may be because only the very serious cases become "statistics." I am not demeaning the effects of the disease on those who are severely affected but only pointing to the possibility that some patients may not have serious involvement and may recover completely without the diagnosis even being considered. Perhaps some people may not even consult a physician for their symptoms of fever and headache.

Of great interest is the finding that, not infrequently, blood tests for the antibodies of Herpes do become positive after a vague illness. It may be that this means that some immunity is developing in that individual because he or she has had a mild case of the disease.

A fascinating aspect of the interest in Herpes is being directed presently toward the possibility that some psychiatric problems may not be the result of brain damage, but may be a symptom of virus disease. Once again the Herpes virus seems to be a strong candidate for the cause of this type of problem. Investigation into the role of Herpes in the cause of schizophrenia and other psychological impairments is in process. As yet no definite conclusions from the work have been reported.

BEHCET'S SYNDROME

A devastating problem of Herpes is a condition called Behcet's Syndrome. Apparently some people have no resistance to the virus and the result is catastrophic.

* * *

Debbie was carried into our clinic by her husband. She could not walk. Herpes lesions involved her face, her mouth, the skin of her shoulders and breasts. There were massive ulcers of the vagina and the anal region. Even the skin of her shins and knees were involved. Her eyes showed evidence of keratitis.

In Behcet's Syndrome the virus attacks many sites in the body at the same time. This type of problem is extremely rare.

The ordinary episode of Herpes occurs most frequently on the lips or the genitalia, but it can attack many different areas. To further illustrate, let us consider two of Ron Roesch's drawings. The first one depicts an unblemished and beautiful family; mother, father, and baby. The next picture shows the common sites of involvement of the Herpes simplex virus. The code numbers correspond to the sites.

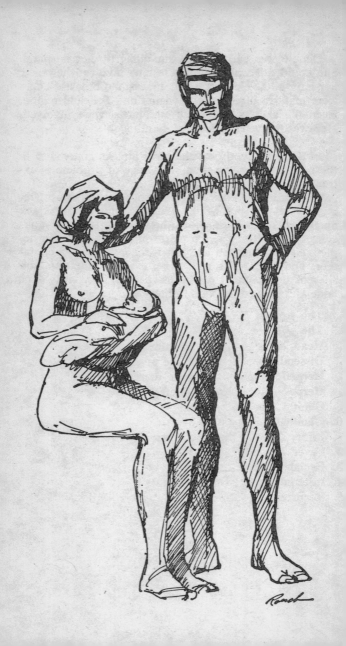

The list of numbers corresponds to the sites of the drawings.

1. The inside of the mouth
2. The pharynx
3. The brain
4. The eye
5. Head, skin, and scalp of infant
6. Disseminated Herpes of the newborn
7. Herpetic Whitlow (doctors, dentists, etc.)
8. Herpes gladiatorum (athletes)
9. Genital Herpes, women
10. Genital Herpes, men
11. Injury (no number, can occur anywhere)
12. Fever blisters
13. Facial lesions
14. Internal genital organs (rare)
15. Recurrent keratitis

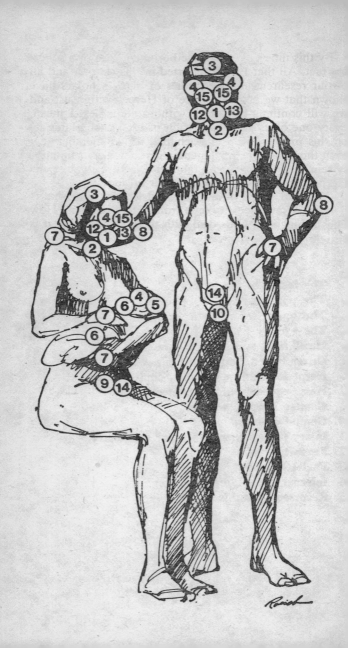

By this time you may have become aware of a sobering fact. All that I have reported in this chapter and all of our research and the studies of many scholars have shown that we have evidence of Herpes within us, and we will continue to have it within our bodies. I mean, every one of us. You, me, each of us. I shall elaborate on this problem in a later chapter, but remember that even though this is a frightening revelation, our immune system is an active and fantastic defense against the Herpes virus and a myriad of other invaders.

Over and over I have mentioned viruses. But what is a virus? Where does it come from? How big is it? How does it function? Let's deal with these subjects, for it is still part of your query about Herpes.

Chapter 3

WHAT'S A VIRUS?

A virus is defined as being one of a group of minute infectious agents. The size of these ultramicroscopic entities is less than one millionth part of a meter. It would take about one trillion of the individual virus particles huddled together in a solid clump to be seen under an ordinary laboratory microscope. To visualize a virus we must use a modern miracle device, the electron microscope, which causes a beam of electrons instead of light to flow over the subject being investigated and, in this way, to form an image for viewing on a fluorescent screen. With this device, the electron microscope, the virus particle can be seen, photographed, and studied.

Viruses lack independent metabolism. They cannot fend for themselves for food and energy but must become a part of a host's actual life to remain viable and to sustain the ability to be reproductive. They fit the definition of parasites because of this dependence upon a host to maintain their own existence.

The way in which viruses reproduce is different from that of other matter. The term used for this process is called replication, which means that a virus is able to regenerate itself not only with genetic continuity, but also with the potential of producing viruses that are somewhat different from the original.

An individual virus particle is called a virion and is composed of three basic parts: nucleic acid, DNA or RNA (but not both), and a protein shell.

DNA (deoxyribonucleic acid) is an acid that was originally isolated from fish sperm and thymus glands. It now has been found to be present in all living cells. The immense importance of DNA lies in its being the carrier of genetic information for all organisms except RNA viruses.

The science of genetics is concerned with the study of how cells develop and how each cell knows what its function is meant to be. How does a cell know whether it is a cell of hearing or a cell involved in sight? This has been one of the great conundrums of genetics since humans first began to isolate microscopic structures. The discovery of DNA is one of the landmark finds in history and it enables a quantum leap forward in studying the destiny of a cell.

RNA or ribonucleic acid was first isolated from yeast and is now known to be found in all living matter. This important substance is also of prime value in life and one of its functions is that of a messenger which transfers information from the DNA to the protein-forming system of the cell. These chemical constituents, the nucleic acid groups, are vital parts, not only of viruses, but also of every single cell in our bodies. They are extremely important in understanding viruses and how they function.

To try to get some organization out of the maze of complicated information about viruses let us sort them into various groups; there are some that may be classified on the basis of the host with which each associates: the bacterial viruses, animal viruses, and plant viruses.

Other classifications are according to their origin, their mode of transmission from one host to another (the arbor viruses and the tick-borne viruses), or the manifestations that are produced in the body of humans. Polio viruses and pox viruses are among the latter group. These cause diseases with nerve and muscular problems.

The Herpes virus is one of a large group of DNA viruses that mature in the nucleus of the infected cell and take over its function. Every cell in our bodies has its own DNA, the driving force that determines the ultimate purpose of that particular cell. It is the genetic presence of DNA which specifies that certain cells will eventually be cells of the skin and other cells will have a different shape and configuration and end up being nerve cells. It conveys the message to the chromosomes that the cells of the retina of the eye are to detect light reflections and are not to try to aid in digestion like the cells of the liver.

Many different specific Herpes viruses exist. These virus particles can cause oral Herpes simplex (fever blisters or cold sores), genital Herpes, varicella (chicken pox), Herpes zoster (shingles), cytomegalic inclusion disease (a disease which is seen in the first few months of life), and infectious mononucleosis (the "kissing disease").

We cannot see a virus except with the assistance of the immense magnification generated by the electron microscope, and this is not practical in ordinary clinical research. We must use other types of testing to prove that a virus is or has been present. Two such tests are important and interesting parts of the research we did at C.S.U.F.

It was in Dr. Jack Bradshaw's laboratory that the confirmation of our clinical diagnosis of Herpes was proven or disproven. If we could just look at a specimen under the microscope and identify the virus organism, such proof would be easy. We can make diagnoses under the ordinary microscope in many diseases but it is not possible with Herpes.

47

In a patient with amoebic dysentery, we can prove the diagnosis by microscopically seeing the amoeba. In one who has a "strep throat," we prove the accuracy by finding the long-chain clusters of streptococci. Malaria is proven by finding the typical alterations of the blood cells that are caused by the parasites. A specimen from the lesions of syphilis may show, under the microscope, the spirochete Treponema pallidum, and this finding confirms the suspicion. Gonorrhea is proven by finding the typical double cocci completely within the cells which are secreted in the discharge of the disease.

In the case of virus disease we cannot with practicality visualize the cause of the problem, the electron microscope being far too complicated and ponderous—and expensive—for ordinary work. Instead we must visualize the effects of what the virus has done. It seems to me to be trying to picture the situation in reverse. It is like the legendary bird that always flies backwards. When asked why he does this, he replied, "I don't care about where I'm going, I just want to see where I've been."

So it was in Dr. Bradshaw's laboratory that we tried to find out "where we had been." In order to accomplish this, all blood specimens were subjected to PHA (phytohemagglutin) testing to determine if there was any reaction. This test records the active level of immunity in the patient's blood. If the level of activity is high, the body is reacting against a toxic invader. If the level of the test is low, the body has little defense capability.

In our study we found routinely that there was a lowering in the PHA levels in the Herpes patients who were tested early in the course of their disease. These patients had immune systems which apparently were poorly able to defend against the onslaught of the Herpes virus.

The particular drug which we were testing had a posive effect on increasing the PHA level and thereby increasing the patient's resistance to the virus. I shall discuss both of these findings at length.

Another series of experiments were run at the same time as a part of the research project. Mr. Robert Settieri is an accomplished microbiologist and colleague. One of his interests is attempting to visualize what is happening when the Herpes virus attacks the cells of the body. As the virus cannot be seen, this process, too, has to be looked at from hindsight. It can be pictured from the effect of the virus on the cells of our body tissues as seen under the standard microscope.

Bob conducted some ingenious and significant experiments by which I was fascinated. Using time-lapse photography he took pictures of what happens to tissue cells when they are attacked by the Herpes virus.

Time-lapse photography increases the length of time between pictures from a fraction of a second to several seconds or minutes. When these photos are shown at the same speed as are standard motion pictures, it appears that there is motion. The prolonged actions of life seem to flow easily.

Bob transferred this process to the microscope and photographed tissue cultures. One still photograph was taken every seventeen seconds. The cultures were of living human cells prepared and kept alive in an intricate manner. Healthy tissue such as blood cells, mucous membrane, skin, and cells of even less accessible organs can be grown and observed. In this culture technique we can scrutinize under the microscope actual cell division and see the chromosomes separate into their component and equal parts. With time-lapse, Bob made exciting movies of this sequence of events. He next added the part of the experiment that makes the project pertinent to our study; he inoculated Herpes virus into the healthy, vigorous human tissue culture. And photographed the result.

49

Shortly after inoculating the tissue culture, the film showed a cell beginning to change shape, to bubble in an agony of turmoil, and finally to literally explode. A few moments later another and then another cell repeated this same awesome picture until almost all of the strong defensive cells were destroyed. Bob's motion picture graphically captured what happens to the blood cells when they are attacked by the Herpes virus.

Remember that the experiment I have just described was done in the laboratory and in a situation in which the concentration of the virus far exceeded anything ever possible in humans. This experiment is of critical interest in the light of illustrating what MAY happen to a very few cells in our system.

DNA VIRUS

Special attention needs to be paid to this DNA virus as a disease agent. The Herpes virus is able to take over the life force of each cell, to destroy the purpose of that cell and cause it to become erratic and irascible in function.

In ordinary times, the virus may enter our bodies. Our immune defenses are such that the Herpes virus seems strong enough only to be able to sneak into the body and subsequently into the nerve tissue. In the sheath of the nerves there are few blood vessels and consequently little blood supply to fight the virus. In that location it can safely lie drowsing until some trigger event causes it to waken. When this happens, the virus begins to replicate.

Because of its property of being able to take over the life force of the cell, the original purpose of that cell is lost and the virus becomes the new despotic dictator of the actions of the cell. The one which is invaded might be a white blood cell whose ordinary function is to clean up cellular debris in the venous stream. That

50

function is lost and the cell becomes an incubator for holding the replicating virus. If the cell is a nerve cell whose function is to detect pin pricks on the index finger, that cell may go into an agony and eventually cause a stimulation of the nerve filaments that supply that particular finger—and a Herpetic Whitlow results. This is the name of the sore on the finger which was described in the last chapter as Jack's problem.

The process is an interactive and diffcult series of events to understand. The illustration of the lake might again help to clarify what is happening.

Remember the beautiful lake with clear water fresh from tumbling mountain streams. The lake was so full that some of the water overflowed and gushed out of the lower end.

Many fish live in the lake. There are trout and bass and perch and even schools of tiny fingerlings no bigger than a minnow. Ten thousand of these little fish swim in one school, a cloud of life that feeds on the nutrients the fresh water brings. By nature, the school wanders in unison feeding in various areas of the lake. Frequently, at an innate signal all change direction instantly to get away from some perceived danger. Occasionally a larger trout may attack the school and a few are lost, but the regeneration of the fingerlings quickly replaces those decimations and their vigor and numbers remain constant.

During this time of well being, some bacteria get into the tiny fish. In the vast majority of the fish, the natural defenses destroy the bacteria before thay can become established. However, in only two of the ten thousand, a few bacteria find a place to survive. The fish generally are healthy and the bacteria are quite weak and have just enough strength to survive until they reach an area of the fish's tail where the blood supply is poor and the defenses of the body are unreliable.

The little fish are trim, slim, and happy. Until the

51

drought! Then the water level falls, the overflow ceases, and waste begins to build up in the lake. The oxygen level of the water lessens and the fish are not as well fed. The acidity of the water changes ever so slightly and the health of the fingerlings begins to ebb. The immune defenses of the two fish whose tails are harboring the inactive bacteria begin to slip.

The bacteria which have been hiding for weeks notice the subtle change in the environment and they approve and begin to grow. As the condition of the lake worsens, the bacteria gain more strength until, in just one fish, the whole direction of its life is determined by the bacteria and the little fish dies and spreads the infection to others. First one fish is lost, then another and more and more until the entire school is threatened with destruction.

If a person can picture a single cell of the body as the tiny fish and a virus particle as the bacteria, one may be able to visualize that the virus can attack and take over the function of that cell and inflict its own destiny on that microscopic being. When the cell is destroyed by the virus the virions spew out into the bloodstream to embed themselves in other cells and repeat the entire cycle of destruction.

In the last chapter I mentioned Ted who had a life style of frequent trips to the Colorado River to go water skiing. His life was vigorous and he was a healthy, active young man. The fever blisters would clear when he was at our university, studying, eating properly, and getting sufficient rest.

There was no difficulty until Ted went to the river again. He would drive late at night, set up a poor camp, or sleep sitting up in his sports car. He would get little rest, be exhausted by the hard physical work of water skiing, and eat snack and junk foods. The usual streams filling the physiologic lake of his life were cut off

52

There was no overflow of water carrying waste. The state of his good health, though it did not seem so, was diminished.

The physical stress on his being caused a depression in his immune defenses. In addition, Ted would be exposed to the ultraviolet irradiation of the sun for many hours. And it was enough. Like the little fish in the lake, so the virus within Ted became active. As his resistance began to be disturbed by fatigue and poor meals, there developed within his body a subtle change. Probably at this time the virus particles lying dormant in the trigeminal nerve began to stir and replicate. This nerve is the structure that supplies sensory fibers to the area of the lips. During a trip to the river a few cells of that nerve were stimulated, but there were not enough virus particles present then to cause any disturbance in the serene equilibrium of Ted's health.

If Ted were to return at that moment to his usual routine at his home and the university, perhaps the defenses of the body—the fresh streams and flowing water of the lake—might abort any further problem. But Ted would not do that. He wanted to water ski. He returned to the harsh sunshine and he "ultraviolated" his skin. The rocks and snags of the physiologic lake now appeared and again he was in trouble with a Herpes lesion on his lip. In a few hours the ends of those nerves—those that supply the sensitive area of the lips—became involved in a typical fever blister.

How long Ted can continue to carry out this routine in his life without permanent harm is something I cannot say. But it concerns me greatly.

You will meet Ted again when the topic of new treatments is discussed.

To summarize, we have seen that viruses are so small that they can be seen only with the electron microscope or detected with chemical tests. These ultramicroscopic structures can take over the life force of a cell, determine the future of that cell, and affect the health of the body of which that cell is a part.

I have told you about the symptoms and some of what we now know about viruses to help answer the questions about the Herpes virus. Another question that you might like to ask is "Am I the only one who has it? Am I alone?"

Chapter 4

AM I ALONE?

Your question, "Why me? Am I alone?" is easy to answer. You are not alone. There is an epidemic of Herpes which engulfs much of the world. It is rampant in the United States, Canada, the countries of Europe, and Japan.

We know that it is an epidemic but we don't have accurate statistics to be sure of the number of cases in any country. Herpes is not a Reportable Disease. The physicians of the world do not have the legal obligation or even the time or the compulsion to try to find out the numbers of people afflicted. But there is a vast epidemic. Of this I am sure.

Possibly one out of every fifteen persons in the United States has Herpes. This ratio is even higher if the figure is applied to the age group of 15 to 35 years. This figure is for genital Herpes alone. Figures from the Center for Disease Control estimate there are more cases of Herpes genitalis than for gonorrhea or syphilis.

In an August 14, 1981, personal communication from the Department of Health and Human Services, Center for Disease Control, at Atlanta, Georgia, Paul J. Wiesner, M.D., Director, Veneral Disease Control Division, wrote to me, "We estimate that there are 10–15 million persons infected with Herpes Type 2 virus, most of whom have latent asymptomatic infection."

Writing for a World Health Organization, one Herpes expert summarized the ages at which the antibodies for Herpes 2 begin to be found in the bloodstream: Ages 0–14, negligible; ages 14–24, 14–20% positive; 25–34, 30–40%; 35–44, 40–50% positive.

The following chart further illustrates the incidence of the presence of the virus within us. The bar at the left shows the percent of persons in whom the virus is present. The lower bar depicts the age at which the virus enters the body. This graph is for Herpes Type 2 virus.

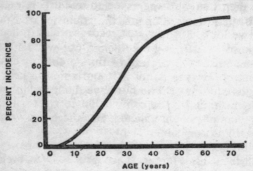

AGE INCIDENCE OF HERPES-2 INFECTIONS

Based on the results of several community studies, a rate of 9% of the adult population infected by Herpes Type 2 virus was determined. If we apply this rate to the 1979 Bureau of the Census population projections for the United States, the number of infected may be placed at 15 million persons.

It must be pointed out that these figures are for genital Herpes and do not cover the frequency of Herpes Type 1. This condition is much more prevalent and, usually, much less severe.

56

Dr. Wiesner's communication makes comments also relative to the increase in the occurrence of the disease, "Many experts estimate that the incidence of genital Herpes has increased rather dramatically in the past 20 years. On the basis of available information, we estimate that the disease now affects from 200,000 to 500,000 individuals per year and that recurrent episodes exceed several million annually."

The communication from the nation's Center for Disease Control has helped to confirm my present belief that an epidemic is in progress.

But in the seventies at California State University, Fullerton, we were not so sure.

It was then that we were asked to undertake a study of Herpes.

When we looked at our past records which reflected the types of cases we had seen over several years, Herpes seemed to be rare. We did note that it had increased in frequency in recent months. As we felt it was imperative to observe a large number of patients in order to be able to properly evaluate the results, we agreed to see 100 patients. Our past statistics indicated that it would probably take eighteen months to complete the series. In order to attract the persons who might be interested in being volunteers, we published small articles in the want ad sections of the university newspaper and in local weekly and daily publications. We opened the University Health Service to the public for this one purpose. We did not publish in the giant daily papers of Los Angeles.

Orange County, California, is a residential area twenty miles east of that metropolis. It has changed over the years from an agricultural center to light industry, another "silicone valley" where the computer industry flourishes. It is generally an affluent area with little unemployment. Many people are highly skilled and salaried to match. We did not expect staid Orange

57

County to be a hotbed of Herpes. We even, half jok
ingly, wondered if the community leaders would run u
out of the area for suggesting such a program. We wer
not sure if we would get any community cases.

There was no need to worry, for patients came fror
everywhere. There were more people than we coul
handle. Our research project demanded thoroughnes
and the numbers created an unexpected problem.

Some folks came directly as a result of the ads. Som
were sent by friends. Others were referred by the O
ange County Health Department Veneral Diseas
Clinic. Many were sent by my friends and colleagues
the fine physicians of the area. Patients were referre
by the major hospitals and from the free clinics.

All came because they heard that a health center wa
trying to do something about Herpes and was conduct
ing a research program into the many aspects of thi
nasty and puzzling disease.

The effect was far more than we had expected and
began to make us realize the magnitude of the epi
demic.

We were not only involved with care of patients wh
fit the parameters of our study, but we also found w
had to do research into all types of the ramifications o
the disease. We could not turn away someone like Josi
just because her lesions were on the buttocks instead o
the genitalia. Walter and several others had Herpeti
Whitlow infections. Must we refuse to see them? Det
bie had the devastating symptoms of Behcet's Syndrome
Should we refuse care? We saw them all. And it mad
our study far more significant.

We even took care of Max, a Hell's Angels type wh
was referred to us by the Venereal Disease Clinic. H
had been treated there twice for syphilis and innumera
ble times for gonorrhea. He now had Herpes. Max als
admitted to having been addicted to heroin in the pas

58

to smoking two packs of cigarets a day, to taking amphetamines and sedatives, and to being a regular user of marijuana, usually in combination with large quantities of beer.

There was no question about the diagnosis. The Health Department rarely makes a mistake. They were correct again in this case. Max had Herpes genitalis. There were blisters along the length of the penis and several more on the scrotum.

But, alas, Max withdrew from our study.

When we explained that we were testing a new drug, one from which we had seen almost no side effects, he declined. Said he, "I don't want to put anything into my body that might be harmful." Well, you win some and you lose some.

One thing Max didn't ask me was the question "How did I get it?" From his vast, past experience he knew fairly well. But you might want to know more.

Chapter 5

WHAT'S A TRIGGER?

A "trigger" is a term to illustrate what causes a virus to begin replication, and the action that results in an episode of Herpes.

Webster's dictionary defines it in one way as, "a stimulus that initiates a physiological or pathological process." It further illustrated by citing that "the sight or odor of food may be a trigger for salivation." The same term is a good one to show what happens in Herpes.

A cartoon series began by showing a bridge with a caution sign saying, LOAD LIMIT, TEN TONS. The next picture was of a truck approaching the bridge. It carried a sign, LOAD, TEN TONS. The third segment showed the truck crossing the bridge. In the final picture a tiny bluebird lands on the top of the load—and the truck and the bridge collapse into the river.

The combined weight was more than the bridge could carry. The tiny bird was the trigger for this fanciful disaster. In a case of Herpes there are many such triggers.

Ted, our healthy water-skiing friend, had a system that lost its defensive capacity when he made the strenuous trip to the Colorado River. The ultraviolet irradiation of the sun's rays was the bluebird for his system.

Anything which cuts down on the immune defenses

of the body increases the chance that some tiny blue-bird will be the final weight that causes a collapse.

ULTRAVIOLET IRRADIATION

The sun's irradiation is a serious problem to people who have a poor defense against the Herpes virus.

Protection against the sun is important, not only for Herpes but also for other conditions. Keratoses (the blemishes of age) and even skin cancer do occur with repeated exposure.

SMOKING

Smoking causes a marked drop in the immune response. Research has proven conclusively that cancer of the lung occurs in direct proportion to the number of cigarets consumed per day; the more one smokes, the greater the possibility of developing this incurable problem.

The majority of patients I have treated for Herpes are smokers.

I am an ex-smoker and, like most doctors, have now come to the firm conclusion that the hazard is frightful. Several events have caused me to alter my life style.

A long time ago, when I was in medical school, a world-renowned professor was lecturing about chest X-rays. He showed the class a film which obviously had a visible spot in one lung.

He then pointed out the faint breast shadows on the film, and continued, "This patient is a woman. WOMEN DO NOT HAVE CANCER OF THE LUNG."

The famous physician was right—THEN. In those days women rarely had that type of malignancy.

And women had not been smoking heavily for thirty years.

Today, women have been smoking for that length of time and the frequency of cancer of the lung in women has almost caught up with the rate in men.

After World War II, 95% of doctors smoked. Since that time we have studied the statistics, read the myriad reports, observed the surgical procedures and autopsies of patients. And quit.

Less than 20% of doctors smoke today.

For several years there has been a strict No Smoking policy at all medical meetings that I have attended. At the International Virology Symposium, which I attended in October 1981, No Smoking was the rule. There was not even a section for smokers. Most scientists, too, are convinced.

Most of my medical practice has been involved with the diseases of women, and I have long been concerned with cancer of the cervix. It has been one of the leading causes of death among women. Cancer of the lung has now replaced cancer of the cervix as the second most frequent cause of death among women who develop cancer.

I am sure that smoking produces these tragic changes because it lowers the level of the immune defenses of the body. Recent research points out that, in addition to the tars and nicotine, known carcinogens, another factor is at work which is entirely different. Carbon monoxide!

The research points out that carbon monoxide is one of the by-products of the flame end of a cigaret, pipe, or cigar. Minute amounts of the substance are inhaled with each draw. Whether the gas comes from a cigaret or from the tailpipe of a car, its frightening action has the same effect on the erythrocytes, the red blood cells. The toxic gas unites permanently with these red cells so they cannot carry any load of oxygen. Without oxygen, the tissues cannot survive.

Erythrocytes are like microscopic wheelbarrows

whose task is to carry the sustaining oxygen. During their lifespan of about six weeks these tiny carriers circulate from the lungs to the cells. Oxygen is carried in the form of oxy-hemoglobin, a loose chemical binding which breaks apart in the tissue where the oxygen is needed. Hundreds of times a day each of these cells circulates to carry its load.

In the presence of carbon monoxide some of the tiny wheelbarrows become like one in which a workman has allowed a load of cement to harden. The worker can no longer add any additional material to the barrow. The monoxide becomes welded to the red blood cell by a solid bond and the erythrocyte can never rid itself of the burden. It will carry the toxin until it deteriorates at the end of the six weeks. Smoking causes some of the blood cells to be so burdened, and researchers feel this lessening of oxygen to the tissues may be more important than tar as a source of trouble.

The carbon monoxide weakens the defensive capabilities of the body and the Immune Response is decreased.

As I've stated, the majority of the patients whom I have treated for Herpes are smokers.

There is an increase in the frequency of cancer of the oral cavity, cancer of the cervix, and cancer of the prostate in persons who smoke. There is also an increase in frequency of cancer of the tissues of the oral cavity, cancer of the cervix, and cancer of the prostate, in persons who have a history of Herpes.

When these two risks are combined, it's dynamite! You can only eliminate one—stop smoking!

TRAUMA

Injury to tissues is another trigger. We see this effect on the lips with Herpes 1, in injury to the mouth and cheek, and in facial surgery which involves the trigeminal nerve.

Blows to the face that cause contusion inside the mouth often cause sores from which the virus of Herpes can be cultured. Prolonged dental work may produce this same result.

Surgical procedures involving the trigeminal nerve are not common, but when that nerve is cut, approximately 90% of the patients develop fever blisters.

Roxanne had a sports car—a small one. She was a good driver and drove the freeways with confidence. One morning as she was driving to work, a truck suddenly stopped in front of her. She was unable to brake soon enough, and piled into the truck. She was very lucky, for her little car slipped under the bed of the truck. The momentum dissipated and the car stopped just before the truck-bed entered the windshield.

Roxanne had some cuts and abrasions and a lot of sore muscles. She also struck her face on the steering wheel of the sports car. There were lacerations inside of Roxanne's mouth but no teeth had been knocked out.

She was observed overnight in the hospital but no serious problem was identified, and the following morning she was allowed to return home.

When we saw her, the main complaint was canker sores. Ulcers of the mouth along the course of the blow of the steering wheel were evident on the inside of the cheek. The Herpes virus Type 1 was cultured from the lesions.

ATHLETICS

Some athletic activity acts as a trigger.

Jock was a graduate student who had been an undergraduate athlete. He still maintained a rigorous workout schedule. His only problem was that of Herpes lesions following prolonged physical activity. Three or four hours after a heavy workout, Jock would sometimes notice burning on his hip region and also on the penis. In two days he would have typical Herpetic sores. Jock denied sexual contact each of the several times we cared for him.

Other physicians have observed similar instances of flare-ups following physical activity.

SEASONAL TRIGGER

Herpes occurs more frequently during the summer. The incidence is far less frequent during the winter, and as one might expect, increases in the spring and decreases in the fall. One explanation that seems apparent is that there is more sex and more exposure to ultraviolet rays of the sun during the summer months. It is also possible that the factors of heat and cold may be important in the incidence of the disease. I have yet to know of any research that looks at this latter issue.

MENSTRUAL PERIODS

Menstrual periods are often associated with flare-ups of Herpes. We observed a definite frequency in our study. Many patients report a history of a relationship between the outbreak of sores and their menstrual periods.

A study which was published by Yale University noted that the time at which Herpes occurred with significant regularity was 7 to 11 days before the beginning of the menstrual period. Further observations of this phenomenon must be made, but many feel there are chemical factors at work in the body that cause such an effect. The great probability is that the enormous hormonal changes which a woman undergoes during the entire 28-day cycle are a major factor.

Hormones, particularly estrogen and progesterone, vary widely in concentration during this time. These variations may be a factor.

One question that these changes raise in my mind is that of the relation between Herpes and birth control pills, which are mainly these same hormones. Why does the epidemic of Herpes correspond so well in history with the advent of the pill? I'm not knocking the pill as a birth control device—for it is the most effective thing that we have—but I am raising the question of the relationship.

Janet was seen in our clinic and the diagnosis of Herpes was clear. There were four sores on the left side of the labia and one toward the back of the vagina. She reported that the lesions had begun three days before and that her next period was due in about a week. Her cycles were very regular and she was taking birth control pills. She also reported that the first bout of Herpes lasted three weeks and that all five subsequent episodes had occurred fairly regularly at about this time of the month.

FOOD

Some physicians feel that food has a particular effect upon the incidence of recurrent flare-ups. Foods high in argenine have been indicted as possible culprits. Nuts, seeds, and onions are a few of the substances that seem to be active in reducing our resistance to the disease. This idea will be discussed further in the section on treatment.

It is important that foods be consumed in moderation. I am not saying that a portion of the foods cannot be eaten at some time. Keeping these foods in good balance is very important. This will be discussed further.

DISEASE

Herpes is often associated with debilitating disease. Maladies such as cancer, leukemia, and the lymphomas are often associated with severe Herpes. Victims of these difficulties are plagued not only with the distress of the disease itself but also with the complicating sores of Herpes. Fever blisters and oral ulcers in the mouth and pharynx are the most common type. These lesions are extremely painful and make eating an agony and sometimes impossible.

The basic cause of the overwhelming Herpes infection is the debility that results from the original disease. The Immune Response is seriously hindered and the virus is free to act almost without opposition.

Until we can find a medical regimen that improves the immune response, there is little that can be done for these patients.

STRESS

Of all the indirect factors in herpes flare-ups, stress is by far the most significant.

There are a myriad of stresses that we undergo today in the strains of life. I shall point out a few.

At our university and at all other schools as well, examination time is a period of great stress. Papers are due, projects must be completed, cramming must be finished, examinations written, grades worried over, and graduating friends bade farewell. There are vacation jobs to look for and make-up exams for which to prepare.

Life is hectic at finals time and often Herpes surfaces.

But there are other types of stress. Money worries, fatigue, how are the children growing up, fear of illness, fear of rape, fear of impotence, success, lack of success. All of these are causes of stress. And all can lead to episodes of Herpes. Another stress that can cause trouble is . . .

SEX

Sex itself, apart from the direct contamination of increased exposure to the virus, may have enough emotional impact on a naive individual, to cause an outbreak. In the next chapter you will meet Fran who had not previously had a sexual encounter until shortly before coming to see me about Herpes. Her story is repeated often.

Dorothy's case was somewhat different but still typical. She had been brought up in a strict family. Eventually she fell in love with Fred. They were to be married. Their relationship had great emotional peaks and valleys. Shortly before the wedding they decided to call it off. But not before Dorothy had developed Herpes for the first time. Fred, too, had lesions.

Dorothy's episodes subsided in intensity and frequency and after six months ceased entirely. A few months later she fell in love with Russ. When they both felt sure of their relationship, they made love. At that time Dorothy had no lesions and no other symptoms. She had even been to her doctor for a check up. She had had no signs of Herpes for nearly a year.

But she was uptight about having sex. She loved Russ and was afraid that if she told him about the previous Herpes bout he would leave. So she didn't talk about it.

Two days after making love with Russ, Dorothy had the sores of Herpes. He did not ever acquire the infection but their love had the insurmountable barrier of a considered mistrust. Their relationship did not survive.

I believe there are other types of sexual problems that should be mentioned. Impotency can certainly lead to severe stress. Plain fatigue for either, or both, sexual partners is a common source of sexual dysfunction that is one of the most severe causes of guilt and misunderstanding.

Herpes is a many-faceted disease. One of the first things most people want to know is "How did I get it?" I will try to explain.

Chapter 6

HOW DID I GET IT?

How did I get it? That's a universal question asked of doctors about every disease. But, when we talk of Herpes, it does have an answer—a strange one. You've nearly always had it!

That answer doesn't help much but it's true. As I stated before, the virus enters our bodies during early childhood. Most children four years of age and older have experienced cold sores on their lips. The cause: Herpes simplex virus, Type 1.

The Herpes virus Type 2 enters our bodies at approximately the time of puberty. Most authorities feel this occurs at the age of 8 to 14 years. The virus can penetrate our body defenses in a myriad of ways; a scratch or cut of the skin, an abrasion such as a skinned knee, chapped or sunburned lips which crack, puncture wounds that might occur from stepping on a tack or a nail, through the cracks in the skin caused by eczema, through the digestive system or sexual contact.

Let us look at our defensive process and what might happen when we sustain a break in the integrity of the skin.

Our skin is like a large plastic bag in which we are covered from the top of our head to the tip of our toes (with a bit of help in the small areas of the mucous membranes of the mouth, nose, eyes, genitalia, and anus).

71

The outside surface of our skin, the epidermis, is dead; that is, it is composed of dead cells which are rubbing off continuously. These dead cells act as protection from minor scratches, abrasion, and friction. They also add a shield and insulation from variations of temperature.

The living, growing, reproducing cells of the skin are buried about a quarter of an inch under the surface. These are usually a healthy pink or purple and are not the color of the exterior tissue. When the outer layer of the skin is injured by a burn or an abrasion, the growing part, the dermis, is exposed. This tender layer is far more fragile than the epidermis. Its prime purpose is to develop new cells which will die, rise to the surface, and become a tough covering. Nature has evolved a system in which all mammals are protected by such a leathery layer of dead skin.

If the skin is injured, infective agents such as bacteria and viruses may enter into the body through the capillaries, the microscopic blood vessels that are in the dermis. Bacteria will cause a reaction quickly in the form of local infection, inflammation, swelling, and often a drainage with pus. Viruses, however, do not usually show up in a local irritation. They enter the bloodstream. From that point any virus, and specifically the Herpes virus, migrates to the nerve tissue and becomes localized in an individual nerve cell.

The reservoir of Herpes viruses in the body is in two primary locations: the trigeminal nerve in the area of the face, and the cluster of nerves at the base of the spine called the "Cauda equina." The literal translation of the Latin name for that clump of nerves is "The Horse's Tail." The nerve cluster, when dissected anatomically, looks like a tail—and the location is right.

The reason for the migration of the virus particles to these particular sites is a matter of conjecture. My own opinion is that it occurs almost by chance. These two

72

nerve segments are somewhat remote and have few blood vessels. Consequently, there is very little of the defensive activity of the blood to destroy the virus particles.

Imagine that a billion minute virions entered the system through a defect in the skin cover, a laceration. These tiny agents of infection quickly got into the capillaries and were scattered throughout the body. They were mixed and diluted in the bloodstream like one drop of raspberry juice in a dish of vanilla ice cream. Some went gliding along in the blood that goes to the spleen, where there is a tremendous number of lymphocytes. There they were quickly rounded up and eliminated by those defensive cells. Other virions went to the lymph glands, where a similar action took place. Still others wandered into the filtering system of the kidneys and were washed out of the body. Other virus particles were caught by the streetsweeper cells which were patrolling the blood vessels. They too were gobbled up. All of the billion virus particles were destroyed or expelled, except for ten. These few happened to miss contact with the leucocytes and were routed by the flow of the bloodstream to smaller and smaller blood vessels. Finally they reached the minute capillary which supplies a cell of one of the nerve filaments which make up the Cauda equina. Along this remote microscopic pathway few defensive blood cells ever travel. The virus particles became a part of the nerve cells. They were able to extract energy and nutrients and to exist for weeks, even months, or more probably, for years without detection or disturbance.

Then a trigger is sprung which changes the immediate environment enough to activate those few particles to begin replication. Soon those nerve fibers become agonized, and a Herpes bout is under way.

An actual infection occurs as a result of a trigger mechanism which initiates a flare-up. Such a bursting

73

forth of symptoms can be the result of one of two factors: increased exposure to the virus, or activation of the dormant virus particles by a change in the body chemistry or physiology.

INCREASED EXPOSURE TO THE VIRUS

In the first basic cause, exposure to the virus, there is a direct increase in the amount of the virus circulating in the body of the patient. This is the result either of exposure to the active, virulent discharge from another individual who has Herpes, or of spreading the virus from one part of one's body to another part (autoinoculation).

Herpes is different from gonorrhea and syphilis. The Herpes virus is hardy and does not deteriorate as quickly as do many germs. Most pathogenic venereal disease bacteria are anaerobic, that is, they live and thrive in the absence of oxygen. When exposed to the oxygen of the air, the gonococcus (the specific cause of gonorrhea) expires as soon as it is dry. Because of this fact, gonorrhea is unlikely to be transmitted by using a drinking glass or wearing the clothes of someone having the disease. It is unlikely that gonorrhea can be contracted from such things as a toilet seat.

This is not true with Herpes. The virus can remain alive at least until the fluid containing it has dried, a minimum of fifteen to thirty minutes. One study reported positive cultures of the virus from plastic surfaces two to three hours after such contamination.

In light of these findings it is easy to understand how we can unknowingly be contaminated with the virus from drinking glasses, public fountains and wash basins, toilet seats, wearing one another's clothes, and touching one's fingers to the lesions and then to another part of our own bodies.

Three examples might illustrate what I mean.

* * *

Fran was 18 years of age and had arrived at our university only a few months before she came to the clinic as a patient. She was a music major who was anxious to become a professional, but she had never been away from home before coming to school. She shared an apartment near the campus with two other women students and found university life to be exciting and a great change from that of being a sheltered teenager.

Fran had dated little in high school and, when the pressure of dating began, did not have the experience, the composure, or the nerve to risk saying "No!" She had had one sexual encounter. Even that one time had been unfulfilling, and now she had Herpes. Her date had not told her until later that he had some sort of a sore on his penis. He stated he did not know what it was but figured it was nothing to worry about.

Fran was greatly troubled. A one-night-stand had given her an infection with painful lesions, had complicated her relations with roommates, put her music career in jeopardy, and scarred her emotions.

Lisa loved sex. She stated without hesitation that she had many boyfriends and had relations often with different ones. "I enjoy the variety!" was her report to me.

Lisa also enjoyed oral sex. Unfortunately, one boyfriend had a fever blister on his lower lip. Three days after having sex with him, oral and vaginal, she developed a cold sore on her own lower lip. At the same time, she began to experience headaches and a burning of her eyes. A slight fever developed and there was a dull ache in each groin area. Multiple lesions began which covered the genital area from the mons in the front, to the clitoris and both labia, and to the forchet at the posterior portion of the vagina. As is often the case following oral sex, many lesions appeared and there were thirty to forty sores scattered over the vulva. Examination of the cervix did not reveal any ulcers. Culture of the serum from the sores revealed Type 1 Herpes virus, and the PHA level showed a marked depression of the body's Immune Response. The fever blister on Lisa's lip coincided exactly to that of the site of her friend's sore.

Randy also enjoyed sex and he played around a lot. Sometimes he had sex with two or three different women in the same week. Sometimes even in the same twenty-four-hour period. He told me of being with one woman four days after she complained of painful urination. She told him there were no sores in the vaginal area. But Randy's Herpes lesions appeared on the top of the shaft of the penis in the exact spot where a urethral lesion of a woman would rub during sexual intercourse.

These three patients represent the direct exposure type of infective process. An increase in the amount of the free virus that is present in the serum which seeps from the sores of Herpes can incite a direct flare-up of Herpes. The process in which the virus appears in the moisture is called "virus shedding," and this is the material that yields a positive culture when grown in the laboratory.

ASYMPTOMATIC CARRIERS

One strange type of transmission must be discussed at this point as it fits into the classification of increased exposure to the virus. This type of problem is that of a person who has no symptoms of Herpes—but who has active virus which can transmit the disease to others. This individual, who may not even be aware that he or she has such a problem, is called an asymptomatic carrier.

Both Herpes Type 1 and Type 2 can be listed under this infrequent but not altogether rare type of transmission. The virus, in these instances, seems to be vigorous enough to maintain itself in certain tissues of the body, tissues where there are many crevices in which to hide. The tonsils, the prostate, and the cervix are three of the most common areas where the virus hibernates.

Basil lived with Barbara, one of my patients. She had lesions of the vagina and ulcers of Herpes on the cervix—but denied having had sex with anyone except Basil. Their relationship had been happy for five years. Each was concerned with the other person and both were very disturbed about the diagnosis of Herpes. He also denied having sex outside of their relationship.

Basil's urine cultures were positive for Herpes virus Type 2. Apparently the virus had been mildly active somewhere in the urinary tract, probably in the prostate gland, and had caused Barbara's infection. During the time I saw Basil, no lesions were ever observed.

He was an asymptomatic carrier.

ACTIVATION OF DORMANT VIRUS PARTICLES

The second type of outburst is more difficult to explain. As I previously described, the virus particles get into the nerve cells and then lie sleepily. They are probably within the cells of the nerves and apt to be within the nuclei of those cells. Months or years may pass without any alteration in this status. Then suddenly there are skin lesions. Why?

The answer to that question lies in the change of the environment which surrounds those tiny virions. This change is the result of very subtle chemical alterations that may be almost imperceptible. A trigger has been sprung and has set off a new series of circumstances and the body had difficulty coping. The virus particles embedded in the nerve cell nuclei begin to replicate, to take over the DNA of the cell, and to stimulate the nerve filaments to unnatural reactions. Even though the virions are exceedingly small, replication proceeds rapidly and within hours there are enough present to begin to have an effect.

My grandfather told me when I was a boy, how, if I would save only one penny today, and two pennies tomorrow, four pennies the day after and eight the following day, and each day double my savings, within a month I would be very rich. I tried this several times, but I never got beyond the fourth day. Viruses, however, can keep up this process until they overwhelm our body's defenses.

Virginia was irritated when I told her she had Herpes genitalis. "How can I have Herpes? I've never had sex with anyone but my husband."

I believed her. She continued, "Doctor Bill, I'm sure my husband never plays around either. It's breaking us apart!" Both of them came to counsel with me and I believed their statements. All of them. Because this does happen.

The Herpes virus can enter the body without causing symptoms. And it often does. It is estimated that one hundred percent of us adults have the Herpes Type 1 virus within our bodies. A similar report by world recognized authorities of the Center for Disease Control states that probably 70 to 80 percent of adults carry signs of the Herpes Type 2 virus.

Let us assume that Virginia reported truthfully that she had had no sex except with her husband. Let us also assume that his report that he had been completely faithful to her is truthful. The factor of probability is

78

that one of the two, or both, have the virus particles somewhere in their bodies. One of the two is a carrier who has no symptoms. Something happened to start the change in Virginia's physiology.

Let us further suppose that, two weeks ago, Virginia's youngest boy fell off his bicycle and broke his leg. Last week her best friend was found to have breast cancer. Virginia's husband just lost his job and doesn't have another one, and the landlord is asking for the rent. Today she started a menstrual period. In addition, the cake she was baking for her daughter's birthday party just fell on the floor—upside down.

Virginia has more than her share of stress. Her physiologic make-up begins to lose its resiliency and worries build up. She becomes depressed and frustrated. Her whole body chemistry alters. Her menstrual cycle causes the hormone make-up to change. These changes are signaled to the virus nestled in the Cauda equina and the particles begin to replicate. Soon there is enough stimulation in those nerve endings to cause a wild irritation and Virginia has the lesions which are typical of Herpes genitalis.

Not only does Virginia have lesions for the first time but also the blebs and ulcers of those lesions now carry a discharge which is loaded with the same active infectious virus as any other type of Herpes. She can now transmit the infection to her husband.

Don was also diagnosed as having Herpes. I did not make the original diagnosis for it was made in the regular medical clinic service of the university. He was referred by that service to the Herpes study, and he had no idea what his trouble was. He had never heard the word "Herpes."

Don was very new to our institution and was only seventeen years old. A prodigy. He did not understand when I began to describe Herpes and to ask him questions. He had almost never heard the word "sex" for he was a reclusive loner. A new student who lived at home, Don stated he had never dated and had not had any sexual encounter. His parents had never talked about sex nor shown much love or emotion with him or each other. He had trouble comprehending my questions about sex with girls and even more trouble with my necessary query about dates with other boys. His love was mathematics, and it was also his entire life and experience.

But he had Herpes. The enormous increase in stress of university life was a major struggle for such a young man physically and emotionally and was proving to be more than he had the maturity to handle.

A similar set of stressful circumstances brought out the lesions in Don that caused the reaction in Virginia's case. The change in body chemistry and physiology activated the virus.

Though I do not have any scientific studies to back up my opinion, my clinical experience convinces me that perhaps ten percent of all primary cases of Herpes occur without exposure to the lesions of other persons. In the cases of Virginia and Don, the diagnosis of Herpes does not fit the definition of being sexually transmitted. Virginia, Don, and the thousands of women and men like them who innocently contracted the initial episode of Herpes, should not be labeled with the stigma of having a venereal disease.

There are a number of viruses that are similar to the Herpes simplex virus and cause "first cousin" diseases. Examples of those maladies are Herpes zoster or shingles, mono, polio and CMV. In order not to be confused as to their relation to Herpes, it is important to discuss them in some detail.

Chapter 7

ARE THERE SIMILAR DISEASES?

There are many diseases caused by viruses and far too many to begin to cover them all. Our discussion will relate only to a few diseases which are similar to Herpes and sometimes confused with it. All the diseases which I shall mention have the common factor of being caused by viruses (or thought to be so caused) and to have a latent phase in which nothing seems to happen except the virus particles drowse in nerve tissue. Some of the problems are often so mild that they do not even let the person who has the disease know that a sickness has occurred. Others of this group can cause death. Examples of these diseases are Herpes zoster ("shingles"), infectious mononucleosis, poliomyelitis, and cytomegalo virus disease.

HERPES ZOSTER ("SHINGLES")

Herpes zoster is often confused with Herpes genitalis and labialis because of its unfortunate name, but it is an entirely separate disease. Shingles is caused by a virus called varicella. (Sometimes it is called the varicella-zoster virus.) It is entirely different from the Herpes simplex hominus virus. However, the confusion is intensified by the similarity in the symptoms and findings.

The significance of Herpes zoster is that it usually occurs in age groups considerably older than those of Herpes simplex virus disease. In persons of more advanced years, the condition can be a devastating source of continuing distress. Though it is ordinarily seen in those of mature years, this is not always the case. I had the disease while I was in undergraduate university. The recovery time in younger patients is often much shorter than in the elderly.

Shingles is characterized by an area of localized pain and eruption along the skin distribution of sensory nerves. The virus that causes shingles also causes chicken pox. Like Herpes, the virus enters the body and hides in nerve tissue, but this time the hiding place is in the sensory nerve roots that emerge from the spinal cord. The virions embed themselves in the nuclei of those nerve cells. Eventually some trigger may cause the virions to begin to replicate and, in turn, to irritate the nerve filaments. The endings of those nerves (where they supply the skin surface) begin to pain and eventually to blister. Extremely localized areas of the body are then involved.

These localized areas are named for the segment of the spinal cord which those nerves supply. Typical segmental distributions are: the sixth cervical nerve which sensitizes the skin below the breast exactly from the midline in back to the midline in front, the eighth cervical and the first thoracic nerve fibers which go to the area of the little finger and exactly one half of the lengthwise surface of the ring finger. The first and second sacral nerves send filaments to the bottom of the heel.

These circumscribed local areas of the body are called dermatomes. Many dermatomes have been delineated and they cover the entire surface of the body. When the nerves of a particular dermatome are irritated by the Herpes zoster virus, the painful rash occurs just in the localized area of the nerves which supply it.

The rash is often preceded by two or three days of fever and a burning of the skin. This sensation is not unlike the burning feeling of severe and localized sunburn. Next small red blisters appear. These vesicles at first contain clear fluid which soon turns to a turbid milky appearance. In about five to ten days the vesicles begin to dry. However, in some persons the healing is delayed and the blisters join together. This coalescence forms large, painful, and inflamed areas.

The pain is often severe, particularly in people of more mature years. In the elderly, it often transpires that the healing process is slow and the lesions persist for months or even become permanent. This type of problem occurs when there is stimulation of the exquisitely sensitive nerve endings, those tiny nerve filaments which terminate in our skin surface and supply to our brain the most important information that something is wrong. When the nerve filaments, called neurons, are continuously irritated by the virus, permanent scarring may occur. Unfortunately, there is no medication that will heal permanently damaged sensory nerve endings. Unalterable pain often results. Occasionally surgery is advised for the interruption of the nerve tracts which supply the affected areas.

The area of the trunk is the most frequent site of the lesions.

Rose complained of burning pain on an area of her back just below the right side of her shoulder blade. The area was almost in the axilla. She told me that for four days nothing could be seen. She continued, "The pain was like fire. It was so severe it almost made me cry. I thought I had pulled a muscle when I carried my grandson around. He's very heavy, you know. He's up to twelve pounds. Well, anyway, today this rash broke out. And there are other areas under my right breast which feel the same."

My examination revealed blisters just to the right of the right shoulder blade. The lesions were in an area about the size of two silver dollars. They were inflamed and angry appearing. Some of the blisters had broken and others were becoming more dry. All of the sores were located in a band which started at the midline in the back and went down and toward the front. There were beginning sores on the lower part of the breast and the upper part of the abdomen. No vesicles were found on the left side of Rose's body. The patient had not lifted her breast or examined her skin in the mirror except where the obvious rash was evident.

The diagnosis was apparent. Rose had Herpes zoster, "shingles."

About fifteen percent of the blisters of the disease occur on the scalp and face.

Madam Algri had been an opera star. In her seventies, she was vibrant and graceful. She maintained her health and beauty with diligence, and, when sores on her scalp began to appear she sought help as soon as possible. Four clusters of blisters were evident through the flow of her white hair and were just above the left ear. These caused burning and some discharge that caused little scabs in the area. There was also a sore that developed on her cheek and one at the tip of her nose. Her eyelid was severely swollen and there was some conjunctivitis. As these, coupled with the sore on her nose, were concerning symptoms, she was asked to see an ophthalmologist in consultation and it was found that there was a small but developing keratitis of the cornea of her eye.

With excellent care no residual visual irregularity renained and the lesions on her face and scalp cleared lowly. The emotional disturbance to Madam Algri's elf-confidence was great as she could not shampoo her hair for several days and the lesions on her face were ar more distasteful to her than to her associates and riends. But she felt distressed—and the feelings of any erson are vitally important and must be considered.

Madam Algri's condition cleared, but she must be careful, for the possibility of glaucoma occurring as a uture consequence is very real.

Two "common knowledge" bits of information about Herpes zoster are false. One is that "If the sores wrap completely around you, you will die." You won't. Even uch a symptom is rare. In thirty years of medical practice I have never seen such a case.

The other is that shingles renders a person immune o further attacks of shingles. It doesn't. But the chance f getting it again is no greater than it was before the irst attack. In this way the disease differs dramatically rom that of Herpes simplex.

Another curious fact is that children can be infected with chicken pox from someone having Herpes zoster, and older people apparently may become infected with zoster by contacting children with chicken pox. However, there does not appear to be much transmission of hingles between adults.

It cannot be stressed strongly enough that grandparents and others who have shingles must not contact hildren and especially infants who have never had hicken pox.

A severe complication of the disease of chicken pox is hat which occurs when a mother contracts the disease uring her pregnancy. Herpes zoster may be a life complicating condition of the baby when it is born.

In Chapter 14, I will discuss some of the new treatments for shingles that will be soon be available.

INFECTIOUS MONONUCLEOSIS
("THE KISSING DISEASE")

Like Herpes virus disease, mono is usually a problem of younger people. The cause is probably a Herpes-like virus, but this has not been absolutely proven. The disease is probably transferred from one individual to another in a manner similar to the Herpes virus: on drinking glasses, by kissing someone who is infected, using someone else's toothbrush, razor, or cosmetics. It can be easily transferred to another person by smoking a cigaret someone else has lit—or passing a roach of marijuana from person to person. Borrowing a friend's lipstick is a particularly bad idea. This advice holds true in Herpes as well as mono.

This disease is characterized by headache, sore throat, enlarged lymph nodes, and fatigue. Severe involvement may cause a transient generalized rash, enlargement of the spleen, and tenderness of the liver.

Diagnosis is made by the clinical picture with confirmation by the laboratory. Lymphocytes that have abnormal shape are found in blood specimens and also a specific blood test may be positive.

Mono usually is a benign disease and the patient recovers completely without treatment except for rest and care of the symptoms.

POLIOMYELITIS ("INFANTILE PARALYSIS")

Polio is a rare disease today. The majority of our superbly trained younger physicians have never seen a case. Not so with the doctors of my generation. In the 1950s there were years when over two thousand cases were diagnosed in Orange County alone. And the area in those days had one tenth of the present population. I personally delivered babies of a dozen mothers who were in "iron lungs" at the time of the birth. One of my professors at the Los Angeles County General Hospital had delivered over two hundred. A terrifying experience for the mother. And for the doctor as well. I never want to see that kind of case again!

In those years the fear of every parent was that fever and headache and muscle pains suffered by their child in the usual activities of play were the herald signs of this dread malady. Jean and I recall vividly when our middle daughter, Kay, fell while toddling across the playroom floor. She was three. When she began to cry with pain in her leg, we were terrified like any other parents. Our orthopedist friend took X rays which proved that it was not polio but a crack in the bone of the thigh. I remember saying elatedly to Jean, "Thank God it's only a broken leg."

Kay is now a doctor herself, a psychologist, but she does not need to worry about the fear of polio for her two small boys, thanks to the miracle work of the two scientists, Dr. Albert Sabin and Dr. Jonas Salk. Their brilliant findings have made most of the world free of the disease. Only in some of the more remote areas is polio still a scourge. I encountered polio once again while we were working at a Methodist Mission hospital in what is now Zimbabwe.

Shamba was seven but he could not walk. Like most of the African children in the Mashona area of Zimbabwe, he was lean and lank with the slightly protruding belly of the nearly starved. A gently smiling little boy, he had been brought to the hospital by his mother. Our examination revealed a marked shortening of the calf muscles in his right leg. There was a resultant foot drop because the large muscle in the back of the leg was stronger than the ones in front and when polio struck, the large muscle went into spasm, pulling up the heel and causing the toe to point—permanently. Walking was nearly impossible.

The first task that we had with Shamba was to build up his resistance and his health. He was very anemic. Iron and vitamins, and particularly protein in his diet, a rarity among the Africans, were given as much as our meager supplies would allow. Surgery was performed by my colleague and friend, Dr. Gerald Downie, to strengthen and lengthen the paralyzed muscles. With training and rehabilitation Shamba was finally able to walk out of the mission complex and return to his home. With his head held high, and a grin of joy and pride, this young man had a new opportunity to become a valued part of his society.

Nyasha also had the residuals of polio. But we did not treat her for that. The 19-pound 6-year-old was starving. Her black skin had turned brown and her hair even had a reddish tinge. There were cracks in the skin at each joint of the body. Her subdued countenance was not entirely due to her fear of the white "cheremba," the Shona word for doctor. She had "kwashiorkor," a severe protein deficiency disease, in addition to the polio residuals which had paralyzed both legs. These children are irritable and unhappy when they have no protein in their diet—and most of the parents are too poor to furnish any. In addition, a deformed little one is almost an outcast. The "Meals for Millions" food eventually helped Nyasha to return home in better condition physically. But she was returning to the same situation from which she came. We felt that she would sooner or later be returning to the hospital for we were unable to help with the basic cause of the problems, the paralysis of polio and starvation.

The virus of polio is quite similar in its actions to that of the viruses of Herpes zoster and Herpes simplex.

88

The difference is that the virus hides, not in the sensory nerves, but in the motor nerve roots of the spinal cord. Those nerves are insulted by the trauma of the attack of the virus and many filaments are destroyed. If enough of the nerve is so damaged the strength of the muscles which that nerve supplies is lost, and muscle weakness and paralysis result.

To this day no treatment exists for polio except that of prevention. The physical therapy for muscle weakness and the lengthy re-education for strength is wonderfully beneficial but really is a treatment of the effects of the disease. A tragedy of our times is that many parents forget or fail for some other reason to insist upon their children being immunized in infancy. Some doctors, not having known the calamity of active polio on the patient and all of the family, do not encourage or insist upon such immunization. The disease, like the virus of Herpes, is still among us. It awaits only the proper trigger to burst forth again. In unimmunized children lies a pool of danger.

CYTOMEGALIC INCLUSION DISEASE

This condition is a virus disease that may occur congenitally and later in life. It is characterized by changes in infected cells. These cells enlarge and contain a prominent inclusion body, a structure which is often temporary and is seen as a constituent of the cytoplasm of the cell. In this disease, the finding of the inclusions seems to be diagnostic of the problem.

The congenital infection is manifest by fever, inflammation of the liver (hepatitis), jaundice or a yellow tinge to the skin, and purpura, a hemorrhagic state which is characterized by patches of purplish discoloration caused by local bleeding into the tissues and mucous membrane.

The postnatal-acquired infection often is asymptomatic but it may produce many of the same symptoms seen in the newborn.

The human cyytomegaloviruses are related to the Herpes viruses in the way they react in the laboratory and by their liking for a long latent period in their attack upon humans.

Some of these ubiquitous viruses may cause the host to secrete virus in the urine or saliva for months. The virus may be cultured from the cervix and human milk. Contact with fresh blood from individuals that do not appear to be infected may produce the disease in susceptible individuals.

I cite this problem because of the similarities of the disease to that of Herpes and we shall discuss some of its aspects in another chapter.

Chapter 8

WHAT IS THE IMMUNE RESPONSE?

Herpes will go away. It will heal itself in varying lengths of time. Sometimes the infection disappears after only one or two days. It may continue for several weeks. Generally, the first infection lasts longer than recurrent episodes.

The length of time of healing of the individual bout of Herpes depends on two factors: the severity of the contamination, that is, how much of the actual virus gets into the body, and—the resistance of the individual to the disease, that is, one's own Immune Response.

We know that antibodies are detected in our system. These chemical elements of reaction to a disease appear in our blood and show up whenever there is a toxic disease process which has occurred. Usually the presence of the antibodies indicates a good resistance to the hazard. By measuring them we can judge the level of the resistance our bodies have to the infection.

Not so with Herpes. Antibodies do begin to appear in the bloodstream about a week after an infection commences, and the level peaks in three to four weeks. They persist in the body for many years. However, most authorities report that antibodies provide little immunity against recurrent episodes.

On the other hand the cellular immune function

plays a much more important role in the resistance that an individual has. Patients with severe Herpetic lesions often have a marked reduction of the cellular immune response; the defensive cells of the bloodstream don't work to defeat the disease. They are not as efficient as they should be.

I will briefly sketch a few of the many cells which are important in the Immune Response in order that you may understand better the extremely complicated defenses of our blood.

I realize this next section is very heavy, but if you can wade through the mire it will help you understand better why Herpes is such a complicated disease and why the treatment of Herpes must be a multi-sided program. To help clarify this information, there is a chart at the end of this section. An International Award-winning film on the Immune Response is available for anyone wishing to view it. It gives an excellent illustration of how the defenses of the body function. I can recommend it for viewing by physicians, college or high school students, or even small groups. Contact Newport Pharmaceuticals International, Inc., 1590 Monrovia Ave., Newport Beach, California 92660.

THE IMMUNE RESPONSE

All blood cells originate in the bone marrow. The marrow produces stem cells which are undifferentiated, that is they don't seem to give any evidence of the kind of cell they are to become. Stem cells replenish the blood with new cells of many different varieties.

After the stem cells achieve a certain development, they leave the bone marrow for other sites where their maturation continues. Some go to the thymus gland and become T-lymphocytes. Others go to the lymphoid tissue near the intestine where plasmacytes have their origin. These same cells develop into B-lymphocytes.

The T-lymphocytes leave the thymus gland and enter the bloodstream. There each cell is programmed to fight one specific poison or antigen. This process is designated as the cells becoming "committed." When such a specific contact occurs between these committed cells and the antigen for which they are programmed, the cells proliferate and become T-killer and T-helper cells. The killer cells do actual combat with the toxic antigen that is poisoning the system. The helper cells become messengers to go where needed—to be the reserves.

The way in which being a committed cell works might be likened to a set of machine-tool wrenches which fit only a very specific size nut. Any nut that is too large does not allow the fitted wrench socket to engage and so nothing happens when the handle is turned. One that is smaller than the socket slips, and no purchase or strength can be exerted to turn the bolt. It is only when the socket is the exact size of the nut that there is a perfect union and enormous force can be transferred from the handle of the wrench to the bolt of which the nut is a part. An everyday illustration of this set of circumstances involves the lug nuts that hold the wheel and tire to the axle of an automobile. In order to turn the lugs, remove the wheel, and change a tire, the socket of the wrench must fit the lugs exactly or nothing happens.

In a like manner each committed T-cell is programmed to respond only to an antigen with a particular molecular structure. Like a lug wrench whose socket does not fit, if the molecular structure of the T-cell is not exactly like the one for which it is programmed, nothing will happen.

A few definitions which must be as clear as possible to avoid getting lost in the complexities of the subject:

An ANTIGEN is any substance whose chemical configuration allows it to be subject to reactions with an antibody or lymphocyte that is specifically geared to its particular chemistry.

TARGET CELLS are those which are infected and are marked for destruction like those TV gangster movie characters on whom the Mafia have put out a "contract." These cells have been entered by a virus or other contaminant or changed in some way into malignant cells. The changes which have occurred to the cells show up in the cell membrane, the outer covering of this microscopic structure. The lymphocytes which are "committed" to that particular chemical change then become activated and the cell is targeted for annihilation. It has become a liability to the body and the immune response is such that it must be destroyed in order for the whole of the body to be benefited.

MACROPHAGES are the streetsweepers of the bloodstream. They attack any foreign substance. It is not a specific response like that of the T- or B-cells, but occurs whenever these cells recognize foreign matter such as antigens, viruses, or bacteria. The cells ingest that matter and then break it down chemically.

IMMUNOGLOBULINS are the big guns of the B-cell immune reaction. These chemical substances become bound to a cell which has been infected by a virus or a bacteria. They may also act in a similar way with malignant tumor cells by interfering with viral attachment to the host cell.

LYMPHOKINES are the chemical substances released by the lymphocytes to neutralize an antigen and to call the macrophages.

INTERFERON is a chemical substance released by the defensive cells which aids in the protection of normal cells.

These are but a few of the conglomeration of cells that work in partnership in the maintenance of our wondrous immune response.

The following schematic of THE IMMUNE RESPONSE may help to clarify this complex subject.

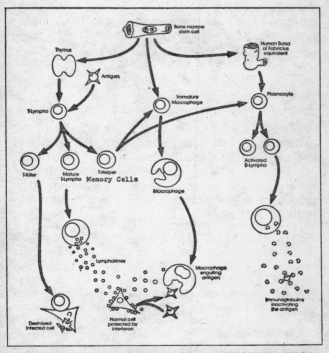

SIMPLIFIED IMMUNE REACTION TO AN INFECTIVE ANTIGEN

Chapter 9

HOW DO I KNOW IF I'VE GOT IT?

Sometimes Herpes is impossible to diagnose. Sometimes it likes to hide. Sometimes it's easy to detect.

When the virus particles are embedded in nerve tissue, there is no sign that the disease is present. None! At this time we as physicians and scientists are not able to detect that presence except through the finding of antibodies which may or may not be present. Even finding those doesn't help much, for it only tells us that at some time in the past, some blood cells encountered the virus particles. Even when the active symptoms are present, it may be difficult to find the sores. This happens when the lesions are inside the vagina, on the cervix, or in the anus.

Your physician and some nurse practitioners have the special skills and instruments to find the areas of trouble.

However, the times when the diagnosis is easy is what I want to discuss. Frequently you can make your own assessment of the disease. You can then point out the lesions to your personal health professional for confirmation of what you suspect. This substantiation of the diagnosis is important, for there are several conditions that are similar and can be confusing. Treatments for these other diseases vary widely and are quite specific.

Before you can assist in making your own diagnosis of Herpes you need to be informed about a few of the diseases that cause confusion.

SYPHILIS

Syphilis is the most severe of all the sexually transmitted diseases. It has four distinct phases: the primary phase in which there is a chancre or sore, the secondary or rash phase, the latent phase, and the tertiary or tumorous phase which occurs years later. Because of its wide effect on the body this disease can mimic many others. Sir William Osler, the great Canadian physician and one of medicine's pioneers, stated that, "If you know syphilis completely, you know the whole of Medicine."

The chancre might be confused with a Herpes lesion. It usually is larger, single, and non-painful. The spirochetes of syphilis can be found in the fluid of the sores and a specific blood test will be positive for the antibodies of the disease.

You probably cannot tell the difference between a chancre and the rash of Herpes, but your health professional can determine which it is. The differentiation is vital to you, for syphilis can now be treated by a specific agent, penicillin, or one of the other antibiotics, which has no effect on Herpes.

Glenn was referred to our clinic because of a sore on his penis. His friend had seen the ads and had heard about our research effort. He thought Glenn must have Herpes. There was a definite sore on the penis. It was a little smaller than a dime and had raised edges and a very shiny surface. But the sore was not painful. This fact raised our suspicions and we did a dark-field examination and a serology. As Glenn had had the sore for several days, we were not surprised when the dark-field was negative. The specific blood test was strongly positive and the diagnosis was definite for syphilis. Penicillin in large quantities treated the condition and the sore disappeared quickly. Treating the syphilis did not eliminate the question of Herpes, however, but in Glenn's case, the disease was not found.

If you have a sore in the genital area, the lips, the anal area, or the skin, consult your physician.

GONORRHEA

Gonorrhea (the gleet, clap) usually shows up by a drip from the penis in men and a creamy, profuse, yellow vaginal discharge in women. There are no sores but urination and the discharge may burn. Your professional can verify the diagnosis. The treatment of gonorrhea also is specific: antibiotics such as penicillin.

Lynette came to the clinic complaining of abdominal pain, fever, soreness of the vulvar area, and a vaginal discharge. She gave a history of promiscuity, and I had the impression that she might be working her way through school as a prostitute. There were several lesions on the labia which were typical of Herpes. These were painful and the labia were swollen. In addition, similar lesions were noted on the cervix. The discharge which she complained about was examined under the microscope, and double cocci inside the cells were seen. Also the culture of the secretions showed the typical growth which proved gonorrhea. The abdominal pain indicated some extension of the gonorrheal process into the ovaries and tubes and so large amounts of antibiotics were given. The discharge, abdominal pain, and the fever cleared satisfactorily, but the sores of Herpes continued to run their typical course.

* * *

Syphilis and gonorrhea are venereal diseases, and it is important to remember that both may also be present in persons who have Herpes. Syphilis or gonorrhea should be treated with antibiotics as soon as diagnosed, whether Herpes is present or not.

VAGINITIS

Occasionally fungus or yeast infections of the vagina will cause a severe yellow or white curdish-like discharge. The cause of the problem can be determined by looking at the material under the microscope. Appropriate treatment can then be undertaken to eradicate the specific cause.

Herpes lesions which are inside the vagina may also cause a discharge which is often more watery than yeast infestations. This condition does not cause pain on the inside, for there are few nerve endings in that location, but when the serum spreads over the labia, outside of the vagina, soreness is evident. In that location, there are many nerves which are then stimulated, causing pain.

Nita was seen for only one complaint, vaginal discharge. Her friend, another woman, told her that certainly she had Herpes.

On examination, the discharge was evident, but only yeast forms were seen under the microscope. No Herpes lesions were found. Culture of the secretions of the vagina grew only the yeast. The PHA determination was normal and the Pap test showed only some inflammation of the cervix. The test was negative for cancer, and none of the multinucleated giant cells were seen.

Treatment of the yeast infection of the vagina relieved Nita of the irritation—and the fear that the friend had mistakenly caused her.

100

CYSTITIS

This condition, an infection of the urinary tract, may cause burning on urination in both women and men. Oftentimes Herpes lesions in the urethra may cause similar symptoms. Your doctor can determine the causes by a urinalysis. Sometimes the condition is more complex and further testing is required. The treatment of urinary tract infections is specific and is based on antibiotics of various types.

Thelma woke in the night. She had to quickly go to the bathroom. When she urinated it burned and there was even a little blood.

For the next few hours she had to go to the bathroom often but found it very painful so she tried to hold back. Because it hurt to urinate, she did not drink any water. When the clinic opened she was waiting. When I saw her, the nurses already had the laboratory specimen results. Her urine specimen showed bacteria.

Thelma was terribly embarrassed when she told me that she and her fiancé had had intercourse for the first time. She was so refreshingly naive that it was a delight to care for her.

She did not have Herpes. She had a set of symptoms called "Honeymoon Cystitis," which is a urinary tract problem caused by bacteria getting into the urethra and causing an infection. The condition frequently occurs following the first intercourse. I was happy that no Herpes was found. Antibiotics, and large quantities of water, cured her distress.

SHINGLES

The scientific name for "shingles" is Herpes zoster. In chapter 6, I discussed this disease in detail but please remember that it can mimic Herpes. Though it is a different disease, the sores of zoster are similar to those of Herpes simplex except that they are limited in area—and are only on one side of the body. Ordinarily they are on the trunk or the scalp and face. Your physician can differentiate between the two maladies.

These conditions, and others less common, make the diagnosis of Herpes more confusing and difficult. Professional assistance is needed and important to determine the problem. With personal examination of yourself, you can be of great help in this process.

SELF-EXAMINATION FOR HERPES

LOOK

Usually the lesions of Herpes are easy to see. Sometimes there is no pain and you do not realize sores are present. Look at yourself. Don't be afraid to look at your entire body—nude. Stand in front of the mirror (a full-length one if you have it) and systematically view your anatomy. Make a note of any spots that you need to ask about. Start with the scalp, next your ears and face. Examine each part of your body, your neck, chin, shoulders, arms, and trunk. Remember to scrutinize the armpits. With another mirror look at your back from your neck to the buttocks. Separate the buttocks so that you can see into the fold. If your breasts are heavy lift them up so that all parts of those structures can be noted. (Women, and men too, should perform self-examination of the breast tissue at monthly intervals. For details of the technique, contact the Cancer Society in your community.)

Examining the genitalia is more difficult. To visualize the parts you cannot see while standing in front of the mirror, lie down on your back with the knees drawn up and wide apart. If possible, this should be in front of the full mirror so that the hand mirror and the larger one can both help. Women should separate the labia and look carefully at the folds and creases of the labia and the portion of the vagina that is visible. Uncircumcised men should pull the foreskin back and carefully note the corona and the end of the penis.

Both women and men should separate the buttocks to view the anal region. If you are agile this can easily be done by bending over in front of the full-length mirror and looking between your legs. If you are not quite so spry a hand mirror will accomplish the task well.

Don't forget to look at your legs and feet. Sores can occur there, too.

FEEL

Feel the areas of your body for enlarged lymph nodes. Palpate your neck below the ears, in front and in back. Often, enlarged nodes may be below but close to the angle of the jaw. When lying flat on your back, with your thighs and head completely relaxed, feel the groin areas. Try to detect any lumps that may feel like a single or even a cluster of grapes which are soft. You may be surprized to find some tenderness in these areas. Don't panic, finding nodes does not mean you have Herpes. But if they are enlarged and somewhat tender, it does mean that you should try to find out what the cause of that glandular swelling may be.

If you detect a fullness in the abdomen, that may be an enlarged liver or spleen. That, too, should be checked out. If the enlargement is in the peripheral portions of the abdomen, the right flank, the upper part of the abdomen below the ribs, and especially in the left side, the chances are good that you are constipated. The most common masses in the abdomen are found on the basis of the patient's constipation. If the mass is tender it should be checked by a physician.

103

If there are sores on your body, make a note to tell your own physician, but do not touch the lesions.

IF YOU'RE GOING TO HAVE SEX— LOOK AT YOUR SEXUAL PARTNER

It may be difficult, but LOOK AT YOUR SEXUAL PARTNER! If things have reached the point of sex—things have reached the point of knowing each other. If you see sores that you are worried about— stop! Hard as it is—in any sense of that word—do not touch the sores. HERPES CAN BE PREVENTED BY NOT BEING EXPOSED—far better than it can be treated. Take a cold shower. Run around the block. Go out to dinner. Say a prayer (and I'm serious about that). Talk to a friend. But don't touch those lesions.

For the next section you might want to refresh your memory by glancing at the chart at the end of Chapter 2.

HERPES LABIALIS

Look carefully at your lips. Burning, then redness, and finally crusting are the hallmarks of fever blisters.

Lesions inside the mouth should be reported and described for your physician. The virus is often found in saliva and so there is probably a source inside the oral cavity.

Often times whitish or gray plaques are seen in the mouth, and are probably noted when you brush your teeth. There is no specific location, but many times they will occur on the roof of the mouth, in the pharynx, or on the gums around the teeth.

If such plaques are noted describe what you see fully, with measurements, color, and location. Consult your personal physician, or your dentist, to determine what is the right course for you to take.

104

KERATITIS

Carefully notice any redness of your eyes. Note pain and inflammation of the blood vessels. If there is any grayness or roughness over the central area (the cornea), immediately report this to an ophthalmologist.

HERPES GENITALIS—MEN

Sores on the penis should be studied and any painful areas scrutinized carefully. Carry out any such inspection in a systematic manner. Any routine is acceptable as long as it covers the entire area—but stick to that routine and you will not miss sections. One routine is to look first at the urethra, the tube that opens at the end. Note any redness. Gently press the penis so that the urethra opens a little and note any irregularities just inside. Next look at the head of the penis, at any roughness, discolorations, or crusts. As I mentioned previously, if the penis is not circumcised, gently retract the foreskin and look at the corona and the foreskin itself. It may be necessary to cleanse the area of any secretions that are there. The important part of the examination is to have good visibility so that if a lesion is present you can see it.

Ralph stated that his penis was sore. He was not circumcised and it was difficult to visualize the area. When he came to the clinic, we were able to gently retract the swollen foreskin so that a line of small ulcers could be seen. These were about the size of the head of a pin and did not seem to be as painful as larger lesions. But they had caused considerable swelling.

Any spots on the pubis or the scrotum should be noted by separating the hairs and using a strong light.

Another aspect of self-examination is feeling for lymph nodes. Swellings that feel about like soft grapes may be felt in each groin. These may be somewhat tender.

HERPES GENITALIS—WOMEN

Self-examination for women is sometimes a difficult procedure. Many women find inspecting their own genital area an embarrassing process. But it is a proper and decorous activity. Our bodies are miraculous in all their variations, and we should enjoy and welcome the opportunity to protect our wondrous life.

I've already mentioned that the most important part of the examination is to systematically look at yourself. Be sure that the entire body is studied. One system is to start at the top of your head and proceed downward. Another technique is to examine the front of the body completely, then turn to the side, to the back, and finally the other side. It can be done quickly but, to be worth doing, should cover the entire surface.

Doctors get many surprises. I sometimes feel that I've seen it all, and then a new one appears.

One young lady that did not like to look at her own body, came to the Herpes clinic. As I knew her, I asked about any problems she might be having. But she insisted that Herpes was the only one. During the examination, I noticed skin blemishes that are quite typical. When I asked if she had looked at her pubic area, she replied indignantly, "Of course not. That would not be proper."

The problem was that she had pediculosis, insects that infest the pubic area and can be cured easily. No Herpes was found.

None of this was particularly startling. The stopper for me was that this young woman who refused to look

106

at herself in the mirror because that would be vulgar—was a topless and bottomless go-go dancer.

Checking the groin areas for lymph node enlargement is also important and is accomplished in the identical manner I have described for men.

As in men, the home examination is much easier and more thorough when another person is able to assist.

Remember that notes are important for accuracy in your report to your physician. I have skin problems, and I cannot seem to remember from one day to the next what the lesions look like. I have the suspicion that you may have a similar problem. I'm sure my patients do. So, like my own patients, I ask you to write down any problems that you see. These lesions change rapidly and, by the time a professional inspects the area, they have disappeared entirely or varied in some aspect. I would recommend making two legible copies. TAKE THE REPORT WITH YOU when you see your doctor or health professional. Give your doctor one copy and keep one for yourself so that you will remember what you have reported and the questions you have asked.

CONSULT A PROFESSIONAL. Gonorrhea, syphilis—and Herpes—can be found at the same time in the same individual. You must have competent advice because, as I have previously described, the treatments of these, and other diseases, vary widely. DON'T RELY ON YOUR OWN OPINION—OR YOUR FRIEND'S—unless that person is a qualified professional who can give expert advice in the care of Herpes virus disease.

I will not advise for myself or my family in medical matters. I am too close to the situation, too emotionally involved, to be objective and to think clearly. Another medical adage goes something like, "A physician who treats himself (or herself) has a fool for a doctor." Perhaps listening to one's friends—or giving advice to them—fits in the same category.

DIAGNOSIS OF HERPES BY YOUR PHYSICIAN

Your physician or health professional should have experience in the diagnosis of Herpes. Make certain that this is the case and, if there is doubt in your mind, request a consultation with a gynecologist, urologist, dermatologist, or a specialist in virus diseases. Ethical physicians are pleased to discuss their qualifications and to seek referrals for you. If this is not the case, run, do not walk, to the exit. You are not receiving the care you deserve. Remember, YOU are in charge of your medical care—and your health professional, be it doctor, nurse practitioner, free clinic, or medical school intern, is your employee. Their responsibility is to present to you what they advise from their medical experience, and to suggest a course of action that they feel will be of benefit to you.

Your responsibility is to question the why of such a proposal, to decide whether it is a good plan and whether or not you can carry it out. If you have not done it before, this is a good time to discuss with the doctor the list of notes and questions which you have brought with you. It will assist in the final diagnosis and ultimately in the treatment.

I always liked to have my patients carry a paper and pencil with them at all times. When a question came to mind, I asked them to write it down, right then, not a half hour later, as it could be forgotten. The patient and I would discuss this list at the next visit. It actually saved me lots of time because I could relate to the concern of those for whom I was caring, and it helped to explain my actions and instruct those receiving that care.

Investigation and care of Herpes is a many-sided problem, and it requires a fine and sensitive rapport between physician and patient. That is one of the prime parts of the medical care. Friendship and trust between patient and doctor is vital and without it, the care may by unsuccessful.

When you are confident in your health professional, and you decide to continue, there are certain scientific things that may be done.

MEDICAL HISTORY

To be certain of the diagnosis, your physician will first take a history of your case. In October of 1981, as mentioned earlier, I attended the International Symposium on Medical Virology. Several of the world authorities on Herpes stated that the medical history is the most important part of the entire examination. Your physician will probably ask many questions about previous exposure to the disease, about previous Herpes episodes, and about whether your sexual partner or partners have had any sores. This information is confidential and it is illegal for such to be talked about. In my office, private and clinic, a break in confidentiality is grounds for immediate dismissal of any employee. This same concern exists throughout all of the ethical practice of medicine, and I urge you to be open with your physician.

Your physician will examine you completely and give special attention to the sores which you point out. As I have related, the sores of Herpes have a typical appearance and location.

Laboratory tests will be requested. These are important to determine what virus is causing the problem. Tests which might be done are: virus culture, blood studies for the development of antibodies, and microscopic studies of the serum from the lesions to find the microscopic giant cells. A Pap test (Papanicolaou's stain test) is imperative.

THE PAP TEST
(PAPANICOLAOU'S STAIN TEST)

The Pap test is of vital importance in the care of Herpes virus disease because it is used, not only to diagnose cancer, but also to find the multinucleated giant cells which are quite typical of Herpes. In my opinion, the best confirmation of Herpes occurs when the two tests are positive.

A Pap test is common, but I was surprised to find that someone as close to medicine and to gynecology as my wife, Jean, didn't know what the test was all about. She told me, that, though she had had fine medical care and annual check-ups, that she thought the gynecologist or the internist would "Take a snip of something," from the cervix. She was also under the mistaken idea that Pap tests were only for revealing cancer of the cervix. Also Jean, and several of our close women friends whom I have now asked about the subject, thought that Pap tests were only used in the diagnosis of diseases of women.

Jean knows of my distrust of some things in medicine and wondered if she was having too many Pap tests like I worry about patients having too many X rays.

I can see that I missed the boat a mile or more in thinking I had explained the process of a Pap to our friends and patients. You cannot have too many Pap tests, as it is only a system in which a sample of the secretions of the cervical tissue is examined.

So, because Paps are so important in Herpes as well as in cancer, I had better reveal more medical secrets and discuss Papanicolaou smears.

Pap tests are simple, inexpensive tests to have done. The doctor with the long Greek name has devised a test that has revolutionized our ability to be warned about cancer. He found that a special microscope tissue stain would highlight certain cells. Further, it was determined that certain cells could be seen early, that is, before they became actually malignant. These are what are called "premalignant" cells. If cells that are premalignant are found we can be fairly sure that there has been no extension of the growth and a cure can be effected by removing that premalignant tissue.

The test itself is easy to complete. A swab or applicator is wiped across the cervix, sore, gums, or any other moist tissue. The applicator is then touched to a microscope slide so that a very thin layer of the moisture from the lesion is placed upon it. Next, the slide is dried thoroughly either in the air or in a drying chemical solution.

The slide is then stained with Papanicolaou's special stain. This type of test has been given the lovely title "exfoliative cytology."

A technologist particularly skilled in cytology next examines the slide and searches the entire surface for the particular cells that are characteristic of being abnormal. If there are any cells that the technologist feels might be questionably different from the normal ones, the slide is seen by a pathologist, a physician whose specialty is the study of malignant tissues. The evaluation of the appearance of the cells will be sent to the physician who referred the slide to the laboratory so that there will be a personal follow-up with the patient.

Jean and her friends were right about one aspect of Pap tests. The vast majority of the tests are to tell the presence or absence of malignant cells of the cervix. But this is not an absolute. The test can be used for any tissue, anywhere in the body, male or female.

The usual test of the cervix is quite simple. It does involve a pelvic examination for accuracy. There are other tests that can be done at home, but I do not trust them and would not want Jean or any of my daughters to rely upon those.

To complete the test, a patient is placed on an examining table, her knees are drawn up and separated. In most offices, clean drape sheets are prepared by the nurse so that the patient may be discretely examined. The examiner dons rubber gloves and gently examines the vulva and the vagina. Some physicians use two fingers for this examination, but I have rarely found this to be necessary; one finger is much more comfortable for the patient and just as revealing of any problems to the doctor.

The doctor or the trained nurse practitioner attempts to examine the uterus, which in the non-pregnant state is a structure about the size and shape of a small pear, about 1 inch by 3 inches. The finger that is in the vagina reaches behind the cervix, and the examiner's other hand is placed upon the abdomen. A skilled examiner can detect many problems quickly with this simple routine. The size and shape of the uterus is easily ascertained. The ovaries' size and moveability, and the freeness of the tubes can be determined. Sometimes fluid in the abdominal cavity or adhesions can be found.

The next portion of the examination involves inserting a small device into the vagina so that the cervix can be visualized. In years past, this instrument, called a speculum, was made of metal—cold metal. It was uncomfortable. I always kept a heating pad in the drawer where the speculums were stored so that the chill would not be such a shock. Today most of the instruments are plastic so this is not such a problem. They can be kept more sterile too, for they are disposable.

A speculum is somewhat like the hinged device we have in the kitchen to grasp the ears of corn from the cooking pan, like scissors in reverse. The two sections can be closed to present a very small surface. After they have been inserted gently into the vagina, the interior

112

ends can be separated so that the cervix is made visible. With good illumination (I get far more light with an old-fashioned head mirror than with the new devices) it is easy to visualize the cervix. Ordinarily, I use a small wooden spatula, like a tongue blade, to gently circle the cervix, the opening to the womb. This small stick is then withdrawn and the small amount of secretions at the tip are placed on the microscope slide which is held by the assistant.

Unless there is some problem that necessitates a longer time, the usual pelvic examination takes about four or five minutes. There should be no pain caused during a pelvic examination unless some problem exists. If pain is produced, the examiner is either rough or inexperienced.

In addition to a pelvic examination, a careful physician or practitioner will also complete a rectal examination to ascertain problems in that delicate area of the anatomy.

As I reported, the results of the Pap test or any other tests that have been completed will be returned to the physician or the health counsellor who completed the examination. Most will contact the patient to give him or her the results of the tests. This is the ideal, and the way it usually worked in my office. However, once in a while I slipped up. The patient did not get a report. This never happened if the report was positive. But even with a negative, I believe it is vital for the patient to know and not guess. I think "If you don't hear from me, it is all OK" is about the most unsettling phrase in the English language. I worry for weeks.

When you leave the office, find out when the report will be ready. Add 24 hours, and if you have not heard, call the office and find out what the results are. Do not hesitate. You are in charge of your care and the office personnel are your employees for this one case. Call to get the results. Your life might depend upon it.

113

The diagnosis of your Herpes might depend upon your call, too, for Pap tests are not only useful in detecting cancer of the cervix, but are also very helpful in diagnosing Herpes from any site in the body where there is a sore.

At the final conclusion of the examination, your doctor will make the diagnosis. When that diagnosis is "Herpes," YOUR work has just begun.

Chapter 10

WHAT DO I DO NOW?

Herpes has often, in the medical journals and in the lay press, been stated to have no cure. I don't believe it.

I believe there IS control for Herpes.

That control does not rest on one specific drug that a patient takes nor on one thing that a patient does. Controlling Herpes is a many-sided program. This program involves the life of the afflicted individual.

One can work in three basic ways to control Herpes:

1. INTENSIFY YOUR OWN BODY'S IMMUNE RESPONSE.
2. ASSIST YOUR OWN BODY'S IMMUNE RESPONSE.
3. STOP DESTROYING YOUR OWN BODY'S IMMUNE RESPONSE.

Number 1 involves prevention. Number 2, good health care. Number 3, actions to stop.

I have taken many pages to discuss the cause of Herpes and its recurrences. By now, you know about the virus particles within each of us, dormant and waiting to waken and begin their fearsome effect on our systems. We cannot rid ourselves of those virions, but we can keep them dormant. That's why the Immune Response of our bodies is vital. That response is many faceted. There is not just ONE way to fight Herpes.

1. INTENSIFY YOUR OWN BODY'S IMMUNE RESPONSE

PREVENTION

Sex

Look at your partner!

When you or your partner have Herpes lesions—no sex!

No kissing if you have fever blisters. No touching if you have sores on the skin. No intercourse if you have lesions of the genitalia. This advice includes heavy petting, making out, foreplay, or whatever name you want to call it. Do not touch the sores of someone else's body with any part of your own body!

There is no middle ground—no compromise.

Be extremely careful not to touch the sores of your own body and then touch another part of your own body. The virus can be transferred from your fever blister to your eye by your own fingers. This is usually the way it happens. Permanent visual damage may result. Be particularly careful if you wear contact lenses. Take assiduous care to maintain the sterility of the solution which you keep them in. Wash your hands three times before you put your lenses in or take them out of your eyes.

Sex, even when sores are not present, is a real hazard. Someone who is between regular bouts is less infectious at that time, but the risk is still present. One Herpes authority with whom I talked reinforced this concern. He expressed his strong opinion in answer to my question "In Herpes patients, is sex safe when there are no lesions?"

"I believe that those who say it's safe are wrong. It's a real risk that people are taking."

Be particularly careful of sex when either partner begins to get that certain feeling that a recurrence is about to start. Those sensations herald the beginning of a new episode and, at that time, the virus is particularly active. No sex!

There is little except abstinence that can be done to guard one person from another person's lesions during the active phase of the disease.

If a man has sores ONLY on his penis, or if a woman has sores ONLY in the vagina, a condom (rubber, safe) is better than nothing at all—maybe. This device is a rubber dam that looks like a small balloon. It fits over the penis and covers it from the end to the base. If it is not broken, there is protection of the vagina from the penis and protection of the penis from the vagina and the cervix. A CONDOM DOES NOT PROTECT THE SCROTUM OR THE ABDOMEN OF THE WEARER, OR THE ABDOMEN, VULVA, OR THE ANAL REGION OF THE SEXUAL PARTNER.

Diaphragms and contraceptive gels afford virtually no protection to the cervix from a penis which has sores. Those devices are to prevent pregnancy, to prevent the sperm cells from reaching the cervix.

If you have to have sex—WASH. Both of you. Before and after.

And URINATE. Before and particularly after.

These activities should be done immediately after intercourse. Remember what I said about the skin being a plastic bag which protects us from many things—one of which is the invasion of viruses? Help that defense in an old-fashioned way. By washing.

Irene reported to me that she had Herpes lesions of the labia. She was correct. There were sores on both labia and the vagina. As she was also having frequent urination, investigation detected a small lesion just in-

117

side of the opening of the urethra. She had never had lesions before and had had a general check-up just one month previously.

Irene had separated from her husband and was lonely, when she ran into an old friend, Harry. They began going together again, and soon Irene had Herpes. Harry told her he had no sores of any kind. Irene had not looked. Neither had washed. Harry had a reputation of "playing around" as Irene stated.

I suggested that Irene ask Harry to see a urologist, a specialist in diseases of the urinary tract. He did, and a culture of the secretions of the prostate gland showed a positive culture of the Herpes virus. He apparently was an asymptomatic carrier of the disease.

In this case, thorough washing before and after, Harry wearing a condom, and urination before and after intercourse, might have prevented the initial episode of lesions which Irene experienced.

Wash

The virus of Herpes is a very hardy one. With careful attention, we can make it more difficult for it to infect us. That work starts with cleanliness.

At the beginning of the book, the doctor washed his hands just after examining the patient. We felt sorry for the patient for it was kind of a put-down. But it was—and is—important.

The virus is all around us; drinking fountains, toilets, glasses, the lips and saliva of friends and family, cosmetics, the clothes of persons with lesions, someone else's cigaret or roach. The virus is frequently on our own hands.

One of the first lines of defense is to wash.

A surgeon scrubs his or her hands for seven minutes eight or ten times daily. Those hands rarely have a lasting infection.

It's a good example to follow. Wash your hands of-

118

ten. Use soap and water. Lather and rinse. Then lather and rinse again. A touch of one finger to a bar of soap after using the bathroom to void or defecate doesn't do it. A real wash is imperative every time.

If you or your sexual partner have lesions and you had sex anyway, urinate immediately to swish the virus out of the urethra. Men should shower thoroughly, being very careful to wash the genitals.

Women should also void as soon as possible and bathe thoroughly. Wash the genital region thoroughly but gently, on the outside. Douching is not advisable, for it washes the natural defenses out of the vagina. It is safer to trust the defenses of the body than to upset the equilibrium of nature with an attempt to launder the vagina.

Protection from the sun

Protect yourself from the ultraviolet rays whenever possible. This is particularly true when you have frequent fever blisters. The best protection is to avoid sunshine. The next best protection is to use some sort of sunshade, a large hat or umbrella.

Some people are particularly susceptible to the sun. These are usually white-skinned persons, those of Scandinavian descent, Aryans, or albinos of any race whose skin is without the protective pigment that is so necessary.

Local protection of areas that are known to be susceptible is important. I not only have to wear a large hat when I'm in the sun but must protect my nose and cheeks with some sunscreen. Areas such as the nose and lips should have a heavy cover (zinc oxide—the white old-time salve is one of the best). I don't completely trust the new screens despite what the advertising says, but they are probably acceptable for areas that are not perpendicular to the rays of the sun: the cheeks,

119

neck, and ears, if one wears a broadbrimmed hat Reapplying screens frequently is important.

Some people have skin that reacts to the sunscreen. If this is your situation, don't continue to use that one, but try another.

The broad areas of the skin are not as prone to develop Herpes as the lips and genitalia. From this aspect they do not need to be protected as thoroughly, but for long-term protection from skin cancer, most dermatologists frown on heavy sunlight exposure.

Perhaps if Ted, the water-skier, had protected his lips well enough, he might not have been affected as badly with blisters. He used all sorts of sunscreens and even zinc oxide. However, when he would fall at high speeds, the water would wash off the protection and he would fail to reapply. The sunscreens obviously had little beneficial effect.

Stress

Herpes is a condition in which stress is a major factor. Treatment of the disease will not be successful unless the cause of the stress or its effect is given sensitive attention.

In our study of Herpes, over 75% of the patients who were taking the medicine we were testing were relieved of their symptoms by the end of the test.

About 30% of the patients who were being given the placebo were also over the episode in the same duration of time. Why did persons who were not receiving any active medicine recover from the episodes more rapidly than would be anticipated in the normal course of the disease?

This surprising result is due to what is called the "Placebo Effect." When someone thinks that he or she is receiving a beneficial treatment, often they improve

Their stress is eased because something is being done that may relieve their problem.

Stress plays a heavy role in the Herpes patient's reaction to any treatment schedule. When stress is relieved, the treatment is more effective. When stress is not relieved, treatment is often ineffective.

Reducing stress in all phases of Herpes is important in order to prevent attacks, aid in recovery, or to keep the infection under control. It is a keystone in keeping the Immune Response high and the virus particles dormant.

Techniques of relaxation are part of a program to reduce stress. Yoga, and the exercises of Natural Childbirth may be routines that you already know. If so, great! They are excellent. These programs help to create in you a sense of quietude and help you to purge the tenseness from your body.

Transcendental meditation and, especially, prayer are even more important in reaching out to a force greater than we ourselves. They are a steadying influence.

There is a difference between relaxation exercise and competition. I enjoy both but don't be confused. I relax and feel meditative after a long run or an hour of aerobic dancing. These leave me inwardly contemplative. Not all physical activity is that way. I don't have that peace after a golf game in which I'm playing poorly, my mind is on something else, and I'm getting beaten. That competitive exercise, though it is in the company of friends and is socially enjoyable, sometimes is frustrating and it adds to my stress.

After I have cooled down from dancing, I can sit on the deck of our apartment and watch the sea pound on the glistening rocks below, or go bird watching and feel the ecstasy of the soaring gulls. I can relate to the gliding, diving pelicans, or the flitting little peeps on the beach as they skitter back and forth, chasing each and every wave. And I can feel at peace and serene, even though I know that out there, out of my mind's focus, await business problems, Herpes problems, and the writing of this book.

A book that I think is an essence experience for me in helping to reduce stress is called *The Road Less Traveled*. The author is M. Scott Peck, M.D. It is published by Simon and Schuster. Though I do not know Dr. Peck, I would like to. I highly recommend his book.

Laughter

Another landmark book that should be read by doctors, as well as patients, is Norman Cousins' *Anatomy of an Illness as Perceived by the Patient*, W. W. Norton and Co. The book documents things like the placebo, holistic health and healing, and "What I Learned from 3000 Doctors." He maintains, as I do, that laughter is an essential ingredient of health, and his statement that laughter "is a form of jogging for the innards" is one I have chuckled over—particularly when I'm running.

Jean is a volunteer global executive of the United Methodist Church and spends much tense time in travel and lonely nights. Laughter is one of the ways she reduces tension. She enjoys jokes and the touch of a friend, a television comedy, books—and looking at life with a whimsical viewpoint. It's good to always remember that from the perspective of history, we're really not so important.

We have a group of friends. We have been together ever since World War II. Most of us were high school classmates before that. It started as a bridge club but now we even forgo that brand of excitement. Now we just laugh together. Some travel the world, some are executives that are on this side of the Atlantic, and some remain here at home—but all plan schedules to be to-

122

gether one night a month. I'm not sure why—except to laugh with each other—and cherish the relationship. This is a community for us that supplies laughter, love, and needed support—and reduces stress. I hope that each of you has, or will find, a cherished supportive community.

Relaxation

If you are like most people and do not have relaxation skills, I suggest you read about Transcendental Meditation and Yoga exercising or review the exercises of Natural Childbirth. These counseling techniques are excellent guides to relaxation. The practice of breaking tension takes study and practice. After many years of waiting to deliver thousands of babies, I can lie down almost anywhere, turn off my mind, and go to sleep.

To do this, first you must get comfortable. Lie down on a firm flat surface. Because it helps give the lungs more space, lie on the left side, with a small pillow under your head. Your legs should be gently straight from your hips and the knees slightly bent. The right leg should be on the surface in front of the left. When this happens, you will be turned slightly toward lying on your stomach. The left arm is bent at the elbow with the hand extending above your head. The right hand is palm down and the forearm away from the body farther than the left arm. All parts should be supported by the surface on which you are resting, not by another part of your body.

Now relax.

That's hard, isn't it? You have to sense where to relax, before you can begin to let muscles be free of tension. So, systematically tighten up a muscle so that you can be aware of it—then let go and feel it relax.

Start with your toes. Pull them down toward the soles and then up until you feel each one. Then relax them. Next your ankles, extend and then flex. Turn your

123

feet in and then out, until you can picture each muscle that is straining to cause that movement. Concentrate. Then relax.

Next your calves. Picture those long muscles working. Tighten them. And relax.

Straighten and bend your knees. And relax.

Now your thighs. Lift your right thigh from the surface on which you are lying. Concentrate on those great muscles fibers doing that heavy work. Then let your leg down again and relax. Pull up your left thigh just a little, it's more difficult. Perhaps just tensions in those muscles will be enough to draw your attention there. Then relax.

Arch and straighten your back. Move slightly to bend to each side. Visualize those broad muscles moving the vertebra. Then relax them. Do the same routine with the upper back.

Pull your abdomen in so you can feel the strength of the lower part, the portion that supports all of the organs of the abdominal cavity, the urinary bladder, and the floor of the pelvis. Tighten those muscles and then let them go again.

Lift your right arm, elbow and wrist, then relax those as you did your feet and legs.

Lift your head off the pillow. Roll it gently to the right and left. And relax.

Remember your face. It takes about thirty-one muscles to frown—so a big grimace—Big!

Then a grin, only about twelve muscles, but big, Big. And relax.

Roll your eyes in your head, right, left, top and bottom. Open them wide and gently close.

If you feel drowsy—sleep for a few moments. Or just turn your thoughts toward your complete self.

Quietly.

And then return to your activities. This process may

take fifteen minutes or even less when you learn how to turn off the stress.

2. ASSIST YOUR OWN BODY'S RESPONSE

There are several activities that you can do to assist the Immune Response to fight the virus and to lessen the chance of flare-up of the infection. Good health care practices are:

CLEANLINESS

The Herpes virus is contained in the moisture which seeps from the lesions of persons having the sores. Any activity that counteracts the spread of the moisture helps to prevent the proliferation of the disease.

When someone has Herpes sores, isolate that person's dishes, drinking glasses, towels and wash cloths, linen and clothes. Launder those things separately. Preferably dry them thoroughly in fresh air and sunshine or in the dryer. Dishes should be washed and air dried or use a dishwasher and hot temperature drying cycle. Don't share drinking glasses. This holds true at work, church, theater, school, and other community areas as well as at home.

Wash and dry your hands frequently, using a mild soap (Neutrogena and Fostex are good illustrations of many; ask your pharmacist). I mean WASH. Don't just touch your fingers to a cake of soap and then rinse. Rather think lather! A full sudsing three times per washing is right. Soap, wash, and rinse three times.

Bathe and change underclothing at least daily if you have skin or genital lesions. A shower is preferable to a bath for there is a better chance of the virus being washed away and down the drain. Remember you can spread the virus to other parts of your own body. Wash your hands after touching any sore, touching your lips, urinating, or having a bowel movement. Elementary school advice that many adults do not take seriously.

DRYING

Keeping the lesions of Herpes dry is an important part of the care. This is a difficult task. You must work at it constantly. Here are some suggestions.

After a shower or bath dry carefully. Pat, don't rub, the areas of the lesions. Use a disposable tissue or small towel to pat dry the vesicles or ulcers. If you must use a towel, keep that separate and launder after each use. It is good to place it in a separate plastic bag until the laundry process. Remember that the interior of the plastic bag may be contaminated with the virus, so only use it to hold potentially adulterated material. Dry the remainder of your body carefully with a different towel. Keep your bath towels apart from those of others in the house or apartment.

Talcum powder is a good drying agent. Preferably it should not be scented, or deodorized, as that may make it more irritating. Just talcum.

If you have many lesions, bathe and dry as above more than once daily.

CARE OF HERPES LESIONS

There are many things that you can do to help make the sores less painful. Here are a few suggestions. You can obtain these medications over the counter at your pharmacy. Some may help you, others may not. My suggestions are not specific but are only illustrations of certain types of medications. Such drugs should only be used according to the directions in the package or, in consultation with your physician.

Pain of Herpes lesions
Preparations containing a mild anesthetic:

Canker sores and mouth lesions
Xylocaine viscous
Aspergum or aspirin in gum

Genital and rectal and skin lesions
Xylocaine spray, or ointment
Campho-phenique

Preparations containing no anesthetic:

Oral lesions
Hot salt water gargles every hour
Medicinal peroxide gargles

Genital, rectal, and skin lesions
Milk of Magnesia (yes, the stuff used as a laxative). Do not shake the bottle but allow it to sit on the shelf for several days. Then pour off the liquid on the top. Using a long cotton swab, obtain some of the thick material at the bottom of the bottle. Daub that on the sores. It will relieve pain.

Burrow's Solution. Use as cool compresses, two or three times daily. It will relieve pain and reduce swelling. Ask your pharmacist about the preparation if it is not already made up.

Alcohol, 70%. This will help to dry the lesions but it may be painful. (It makes me hurt to think about it.)

127

Witch hazel. A drying substance that is good but it has the oily disadvantages of ointments.

SPECIAL PROBLEMS OF CARE FOR WOMEN

Washing the vulva with gentle soap is good care. Douching is not! There is hardly any circumstance where a douche is indicated. This fact is especially true in Herpes, for douching spreads the infection.

There are natural friendly bacteria in the vagina. These are called the Lactobacillae or Doderlein bacillae. They are supposed to be there. Their function is to cleanse and protect that structure. Douching washes away those defenses and allows the yeasts and unfriendly bacteria to grow. Despite the TV and magazine ads, don't douche. Particularly if you have Herpes.

Controlling menstrual flow is sometimes difficult. If you have genital Herpes but do not have lesions in the vagina, tampons are best. If the lesions are inside the vagina or on the cervix but not outside, external pads should be used. If the sores are in both areas, use whichever is most comfortable, but remember to change frequently and gently.

If you have severe involvement, don't wear any sanitary napkin but protect yourself with a loose, soft towel which can be easily laundered as I previously suggested. Opened up, disposable baby diapers are inexpensive, soft, and absorbent. They are sterile and can be pinned inside loose-fitting men's shorts.

Urination often is a problem when the lesions involve the urethra. Usually the extent of the difficulty is mild pain or discomfort. However, if there are many sores, the urine, when it passes over the lesions, causes a mean pain. The following are suggestions for help of this difficult situation.

Rinse the vulva after voiding or having a bowel

movement with clear, tepid water. This can be done while sitting on the toilet. Some homes are equipped with a bidet and this is an excellent help. Remember to clean the toilet seat or the bidet thoroughly after use. Please make certain that the water is tepid (not hot or cold).

If the above does not make it easier and pain is still a problem, urinating while standing in the shower is perfectly all right, even if a little unladylike. A help is to gently separate the lips of the vagina so that the urine may flow freely. Continued pain of this same type may be relieved by kneeling in the bathtub, spreading your knees as much as possible and voiding. Another position is that of lying on your back (please warm the tub first with some hot water), pulling your knees up and apart. This latter technique is particularly useful if the lesions are in front of the urethra. Cleanse the tub or shower after such use.

LINGERIE

Women who have genital Herpes lesions should not wear tight lingerie. The acrylic fiber bikinis, panties, briefs and girdles—and pantyhose—are a big help in making Herpes worse. Wear only materials that absorb moisture such as cotton.

Panties with cotton liners are better than all-acrylic ones, but still the area covered by the cotton insert is too small. In addition, often the liner itself is covered by a layer of acrylic so that the effect of the absorption of the moisture is lost. The wetness is still held in the area of the vulva.

Better than either of the above is to wear a long skirt—and nothing at all underneath.

It is important for the secretions from the vagina, as well as from the Herpes sores, to have a chance to dry.

Polyester lingerie and skintight pants prevent this. Wear only loose clothing.

At night, too! Wear nothing, or at least nothing tight. No panties or bikinis under a nightgown. I don't understand why many women have been taught that they must tightly cover the vulva at night. This is an error for the secretions from the vagina should be allowed to dry. Borrow a male friend's cotton boxer shorts if you must wear something. Better still, pamper yourself with a lovely long gown, as frilly as you wish— but nothing underneath.

SPECIAL PROBLEMS OF CARE FOR MEN

Shorts for men

Men who have genital lesions should wear loose cotton boxer shorts. Jockey shorts and acrylic materials keep perspiration and moisture in the area (also the extra heat to the snugged up scrotum decreases fertility). Tight jeans are a "no no." Anything that prevents the moisture of the sores from drying up helps to keep the virus active. So don't wear tight pants! Particularly don't wear air-tight pants.

SPECIAL PROBLEMS OF CARE FOR BOTH WOMEN AND MEN

Care of the anal region

When there are lesions of the anus, having a bowel movement may be painful. Cleanse the area gently before the movement using a cotton pledget, tepid water, and mild soap. Prevent constipation by having bran in your food and much water daily. Softening agents and gentle laxatives may be used as needed to maintain regularity. Burrow's solution may be used in this area of the anatomy also.

Exercise is important in the maintenance of good health. As much as you can do. I run regularly three or four days a week and go three or four miles. My wife, Jean, carries out a similar routine but doesn't go as far. We play golf often and ocean swim almost daily (we live on the shore). Together, we have an aerobic dance class twice weekly—for a full hour each. Jean is a dancer and that is her athletic expertise. I sort of hop around vigorously. But it's great to work out to the full.

Each person should do whatever he or she is able. If you have a bad heart, you cannot do as much. If you have a broken leg, you must adjust for that and exercise with trunk and arms. Exercise with a friend or with TV. Do what your body permits you to do.

Exercise is vital—and vitalizing. But only if it is done regularly several times per week. Ted would only exercise every couple of weeks and for him it was exhausting. Jean and I, who are old enough (and more), to be Ted's parents, exercise almost daily and it's exhilarating. If we miss for two weeks, or even for a few days, our whole physiology mirrors that loss and we feel lousy. If we couple that loss with emotional tension, our whole beings are changed. There is a lack of physical endurance, sore muscles, headache, and even uncharacteristic shortness and crabbiness with each other.

So we exercise in every way possible. We often walk to the grocery store and down town. It just takes fifteen minutes. It's five minutes by car plus five minutes to park. Find a similar situation in your lifestyle.

I climb stairs whenever possible. It is one of the best exercises known. Start with one flight and work up gradually to six or more flights per day. You will be amazed at how your stamina increases. One of the many things I laughed about at the university was to watch the big bull athletes standing among the crowd of people on the second floor, waiting for the elevator, so they could ride down one flight—in order to go to the gymnasium for their workouts.

Chair- or bed-bound persons can work out exercise programs that are beneficial for their health too. Check with a rehabilitationist. The last time I was in a 10-K run, many runners finished ahead of me—and one was in a wheel chair.

HERPES-RELATED FOODS

As I mentioned in Chapter 2, certain foods are troublesome. Some amino acids work against the Immune Response. Others have the opposite effect.

Lysine is a substance that stimulates the body's resistance to the disease and argenine is a chemical that works just the reverse. Diets that are high in lysine and low in argenine are helpful in resisting the disease. Though this research has not been proven to my satisfaction as yet and the several papers I have read on the subject do not cite any double-blind studies, I still advise such a regime.

Recommended foods that are high in lysine (arranged in order of decreasing percentages of that amino acid) are:

> **Goat's milk**
> **Cow's milk and milk products**
> **Figs**
> **Yeast**
> **Peaches**
> **Fish**
> **Chinese bean sprouts**
> **Fowl**
> **Beef**
> **Tomatoes**

        Beans
        Turnips
        Dates
        Egg whites
        Asparagus
        Spinach

   The high argenine foods which should be avoided
(these are arranged in decreasing order) are:

            Nuts
                    Macadamia
                    Walnuts
                    Brazil
                    Almonds
                    Pecans
                    Cashews
            Seeds, sesame, and buckwheat
            Onions
            Coconut
            Hemp or canabis
            Peanuts or peanut butter
            Cabbage
            Carob
            Cocoa

   L-Lysine capsules or tablets, 500 mgm., can be obtained without prescription and one or two per day as-
sures an adequate supplement of this amino acid. One
or two capsules three times daily is recommended when
a person has active Herpes lesions.
   Some physicians advise adding Vitamin C, 100
mgm., twice daily, and Bioflavinoids 500 mgm., twice
daily, in addition.

OTHER FOODS

Natural foods are important in the diet. Fresh fruit is far more healthful than junk foods—and less expensive. An apple or an orange is vastly superior to a candy bar for general nutrition—and the nuts and chocolate are a Herpes trigger for many people. Steamed or raw carrots are cheaper and more nutritious than french fries or potato chips, which have been fried in fat and salted.

Diets should be low in sugar and fat but high in protein. An excellent book that may be hard to find is one by Elizabeth Stead, entitled *Low Fat Cookery*. The recipes are delicious and low in fats and oils. The ingredients can be purchased in a supermarket. This book is one of those things that occurs in life that changes a lifestyle. It certainly changed my eating habits for the better.

I am very much concerned about the chemicals that we put in our water, and on—and in—our foods. What are those pesticides and fumigants doing to our Immune Response? For certainly they are entering our systems. I'm terrified of what the economics of food preservation is doing, through chemicals, to the exceedingly delicate chromosomes of our children and grandchildren. These effects will not be known, or probably even suspected, until our generation is long gone. The answer to the question will not be known for thirty years. We won't know until the two- and three-year-olds of today, whose chromosomes are possibly being damaged, have grandchildren of their own. In the meantime, use naturally grown fruits and vegetables.

FIBER

Fiber in our diet—or as my mother used to say, "roughage"—is simple but of incalculable value. A natural food diet is higher in fiber but it may not be high enough. During our years in Africa, we saw many diseases, but problems of stomach ulcers and appendicitis are diseases of the developed countries, and we saw none during that time. The diet there is very high in "roughage." In the developed countries, we cannot get enough fiber in our usual diet of many refined foods, so I recommend to my patients that they purchase "Miller's Bran" at the health food store. It is inexpensive even though we originally pay the miller to remove it from the grain and then we have to buy it back again! The supermarkets have big brand names that have refined even this product. Look for bulk bran. Bran, two tablespoons per day added to foods (breakfast cereal, soups, salads etc.) together with water (at least four 8-ounce glasses per day) is vital in a healthful dietary regime.

Even the water should be considered carefully. In our home, Orange County, California, so much sodium and phosphates have leached into the underground supply that the water cannot be used by people on low-sodium diets. If the water in your area is so toxified, I advise pure bottled water be used for drinking and cooking.

The combination of bran and water will regulate your intestinal tract, and will carry away much of the waste—and many of the virus particles.

3. STOP DESTROYING YOUR BODY'S RESPONSE

SMOKING

You've probably already guessed my advice about smoking. Quit!

This advice is given because of my great concern over

the symbiotic relationship between two hazards: smoking and Herpes.

So, I have to say seriously, quit smoking.

The carrying out of this instruction is often hard, for smoking is a difficult addiction to overcome. If you think I should have used the word "habit" you are wrong. A habit does not alter one's physiology, an addiction does. That smoking changes one's physiology is abundantly shown in the cough that smokers have, in the mucous which they cough up, and in the lack of cilia, tiny defensive hairs that sweep foreign matter from the air passages.

I stopped smoking when I became really convinced that smoking shortened my life expectancy. The facts were available to me.

But often people do not have enough information to achieve that amount of determination. There are other helps.

Pick out a day when you decide to quit. It may be one day one month, or one week from right now. Mark that day on your calendar. Tell your friends and ask for their help. Particularly tell your smoking relatives and friends. Ask them not to offer you a cigaret, cigar, or whatever. You might be surprised, one may want to join in your effort. It's vastly easier for two or more than it is for one alone.

Ask your non-smoking friends for help too. Many of them may have previously stopped and might have had the same problems and reactions that you will experience.

On the day of decision, do it! Stop! Many of you will be surprised to find your psyche and body is ready to stop, and it will be easy. Others will have difficulty.

Don't let down. Don't take even one cigaret on the basis of your inner mind telling you to cut down a little at a time. That's a nearly impossible method of quitting.

Go for a walk. I'm serious. Start some exercise.

Walking is one of the good activities. Only a half block at first. You will huff and puff. But continue. After three days, jog the block and walk back. It won't be as hard as the first day. After three days increase the trip to three blocks and then to four. DO NOT GO FASTER THAN INCREASING ONE BLOCK EVERY THREE DAYS! You will find that your huffing and puffing is less each day. You will begin to notice that you don't want a cigaret as much.

Don't give up. Gradually increase your activity until you can walk or jog two miles without stopping. By then you will have the problem beaten—and you will find your endurance better AND YOUR HEALTH IMPROVED.

Remember that it takes time. Those little wheelbarrows with the load of carbon monoxide don't disappear overnight. It takes about six weeks before all the red blood cells have deteriorated and new ones are free to carry their load of pure oxygen. And your Immune Response will have a new ally—you.

When you stop smoking, your appetite will probably increase because food will once again taste good, better than it has in years. The exercise program will compensate for the increased calories. BUT YOU MUST CONTINUE THE EXERCISE—DAILY.

So stop smoking. It is important for your general health. When your general health is better, the Immune Response is improved and there is a definite defense against Herpes.

THE PILL

Another of my concerns is birth control pills. What is the factor of the pill in Herpes? Some authorities say that the pill protects against the disease. I'm not at all convinced. Why, in the space of history, has the epidemic of Herpes coincided so closely with that of the

137

advent of this pill? (The pill came into general use in the fifties and sixties. Herpes began to be common in the sixties and seventies.) A second part of the question is how are the vast physiological changes that occur in a woman's body when she is taking the pill, related to Herpes?

I have no quarrel at all about its function, for the pill is the most effective contraceptive available. My concern is with the manner in which it acts and what the long term results of continued use may be. I have prescribed the pill for many years but always with a sense of uneasiness. I no longer prescribe it for more than two years at one time, and never for anyone over the age of thirty. My patients who are on that type of birth control must have a Pap test every six months.

The pill causes a general change in a woman's physiology: there is an alteration in the hormonal rhythm in her body, an increase in mucous secretions of the cervix and vagina, and breast and uterus changes. Skin and hair variations are noted by many observers. Weight control and water retention are often problems.

These physiological changes cause me to wonder if there are not other difficulties that may exist. Our research raised the question but a study of 100 patients, only half of whom were women, is not nearly large enough to draw conclusions about data involving millions of persons. Two worries related to Herpes persist: the increase in moisture of the vaginal area in women who are on the birth control pills may make it easier for the virus to become established in the body, and, the timing of the Herpes epidemic which follows so closely the wide use of the pill.

I do not have hard data upon which to base rigid advice. You must make up your own mind, but if I were your father who loved you, as well as your gynecologist who cared for you, I would hope that you would use some other means of contraception.

In this chapter I have included some of the suggestions that I give my patients. Your physician or health professional undoubtedly has others. Be sure to ask your doctor or nurse for advice and for their experience in treating Herpes. As I said before, you are paying them for their information. If you are not given the benefit of their explanations, and a chance to ask as many questions as you wish, you are being short-changed. A doctor is not all-knowing. Some are inexperienced in Herpes, others have greater knowledge, but each of us can only be effective if our patients understand what he or she is instructed to do—and why! I am referring to your relationship with the super-specialist or the newest intern, to the wise family physician, and to every nurse whose responsibility is patient care and patient education.

In this chapter I have advised what to do now. In the next, we will deal with what should NOT be done.

Chapter 11

WHAT SHOULD I NOT DO NOW?

There is an old medical adage that states whenever we find that a disease has a myriad of treatments and that every physician seems to have his or her own "cure," we can be fairly sure that there is no single therapy. It once was this way for the treatment of syphilis. Now we have one specific treatment, penicillin. It still is this way for Herpes. There are many treatments. Most are helpful but some may be ineffective, others risky, and some harmful. The following discussion is about those treatments that may still be in use that, in my opinion, are not desirable.

STEROIDS

Cortisone or hydrocortisone (steroids) often cause Herpes lesions to spread. These drugs cause softening of the tissues, increased moisture, and consequently, an opposite effect from that which is desired.

I list this problem first not because of the severity of the reaction but because of the recent approval by the Food and Drug Adminstration which allows steroid ointments and salves to be sold over the counter. The FDA has continued to hold back a medication which could be effective in Herpes but has released for general use a class of medications which may make the disease worse.

Please understand what I am saying. Cortisone and hydrocortisone are wonder drugs and are of immense value in the treatment of many diseases—but their action is wrong for Herpes.

I make one exception to this rule. Keratitis may be treated with steroids which are used with an antiviral. However, the tissue of the cornea is quite different from that of the skin.

Such drugs as hydrocortisone ointment, cream, or lotion, cortisone ointments, creams, or lotion or any combination containing these drugs should not ordinarily be used for Herpes. I am concerned that you will hear on TV ads or see in the magazines that an ointment which contains one of these steroids will "Cure skin disease." Medications containing these substances or having the designation "HC" or "C" as part of the label will probably flood the market and be purchased by unsuspecting sufferers of Herpes labialis or genitalis.

Gabrielle's friend gave her some ointment that would "cure her fever blister." She used it faithfully four times a day. By the end of the week the lesion had spread onto her cheek and into her mouth, where there were many canker sores that had not been present before. Her friend had told her it would "do the trick for it had cortisone in it."

Unfortunately for Gabrielle the trick was a Halloween type, for the lesions had spread to the extent that Herpes was present throughout her mouth and pharynx. We were able to culture the Herpes virus from those tissues.

My concern with this type of case is that the pharynx can become a permanent reservoir of the virus, and Gabrielle could become an asymptomatic carrier of the disease.

Two things to learn from this case. One, do not use steroids on lesions of Herpes. Two, do not take the advice of someone else or use their medicine. That type of friendship can cause serious trouble.

READ THE LABEL ON MEDICINE YOU PURCHASE FOR HERPES. IF IT HAS CORTISONE OR HYDROCORTISONE, CONSULT YOU PHYSICIAN BEFORE USING IT.

SMALLPOX VACCINATION

For several years, some physicians have advocated giving multiple smallpox vaccinations for treatment and prevention of Herpes.

A miracle has occurred and smallpox has now been eliminated from the world by means of vaccination. The theory is that, by making a vaccine of the serum of a disease that is a first cousin to smallpox, immunity may be transmitted and the Immune Response built up. This theory has worked in a marvelous manner in smallpox.

The idea was proposed that, if the vaccination worked so well in smallpox, perhaps it would work also with Herpes, as the viruses are distant cousins.

Great theory but unfortunately, it doesn't work. Research studies have not proved it to be effective, and the papers I have read, do not show more benefit than would be expected from the Placebo Effect.

I can often find persons who were "cured of Herpes" after many vaccinations. As it is the usual characteristic of the disease to get better after several bouts of the infection, judging the effectiveness of a treatment by the result with one individual is not really valid. Major double-blind studies have failed to prove any consistent effectiveness of multiple smallpox vaccinations.

Unfortunately, there is one rare hazard associated with multiple vaccinations. It is a condition in which the single vaccination spreads to become a generalized infection. Instead of one vaccination spot on the arm, there are dozens, all over the body.

Janet had had Herpes for four months and there were multiple sores in the genital area whenever the bouts occurred. She was seen by a "professional" who recommended smallpox vaccinations weekly for twelve weeks. It was stated that the treatment would "cure the Herpes." The charge was several hundred dollars, in advance.

Janet decided to start the treatments and received three vaccinations. At that time the Herpes broke out again. Soon the Herpes sores also became infected with the virus of the vaccination and there were new lesions in many parts of her body.

In desperation Janet went to the emergency room of a fine hospital. When a colleague of mine saw Janet for the first time, she was seriously ill. Hospitalization in isolation was required and there was great concern for her life before she recovered from the condition called generalized vaccinia. Janet's bouts of Herpes continued.

X-RAY IRRADIATION

Few physicians today advise X-ray therapy for Herpes. It was once used as a method of treatment. I mention it only to condemn it because of the potential danger of radiation contamination to the patient.

ULTRAVIOLET LIGHT IRRADIATION

A popular treatment a few years ago was irradiation of the lesions with ultraviolet light. My previous comments have been legion on the hazards of the ultraviolet rays of the sun.

Myriam came to the clinic for treatment of her Herpes lesions. Upon examination, I found several genital sores on the labia and the forchet. They were very painful.

In addition, I found sunburn!

Sunburn in Southern California is not ordinarily startling. But this was. It was upside down! It began on the inner surfaces of the patients's mid thighs and went upward to the vulva and labia and abdomen. It jumped then to the undersurfaces of her breasts and even to the area under the chin and the lobes of her ears.

Myriam had seen a health advisor and had been recommended to have ultraviolet light treatments. The advisor had begun therapy and apparently Myriam had been overcooked. During the procedure she was lying on her back with her knees drawn up and separated. The lamp had been placed between her legs. Fortunately, her eyes had been covered or she might have suffered a critical burn of the cornea. As it was, her only serious problem was her bottom and breasts. Painful but not permanent.

We treated both the sunburn and the Herpes. Ultraviolet irradiation can be hazardous. In addition, most authorities do not feel that a good case can be made for its use as being an effective means of treatment of Herpes.

PHOTOINACTIVATION WITH DYES

Another colorful treatment is the use of dyes and photoinactivation. Ther original concept is that neutral red dye in the presence of light alters the character of the virus so that it is not so pathogenic. This doesn't work, but a few years ago the treatment was popular,

145

and as I said, colorful. The patient's lesions were painted with red dye (and other colors), and then exposed to lights which activated the dye. We have had patients with red bottoms, green bottoms, and blue bottoms come into our clinic. I kept awaiting someone with all three together but, alas, that did not happen.

Floyd was an interesting young man of 22 years. He was referred to the clinic from one of the very fine local hospitals. He had been treated elsewhere and had just moved to the area. None of the local physicians had cared for him. When he entered and was examined, he told me of the Herpes which had been recurring for about four months. His examination revealed a scarlet red penis, scrotum, and upper thighs. It was the residual of the neutral red dye program of therapy. The lesions had been present for ten days and were drying up. This is the usual course of the disease so no treatment was instituted at that time.

Floyd returned about one month later when his lesions broke out again. This time he was entered into the study. Unfortunately we found out later that he received the placebo, so no comparison could be achieved in his case. Even without any treatment (the placebo being of no value), his sores cleared in the same length of time as they had when he was painted red.

Few physicians now advocate the treatment, for there is concern that the dye in the skin may lead to malignant changes. I have never seen such an alteration but some report that the potential is there.

These are but a few of the many different therapies that have been tried in the past. There are treatments that physicians are utilizing today that are of benefit. The next chapter deals with those.

Chapter 12

WHAT CAN MY DOCTOR DO?

This chapter is difficult to write, for the things which your doctor can do are limited. Those things are limited by lack of effective medications. In the United States, those treatments are restricted by the Food and Drug Administration. Medications which are beneficial have not been authorized for use despite the fact that at least one such is being actively prescribed and used without side effects in 51 other nations. That medication and others will be described in the chapter titled "What's in the Future for Treatment." The drug which we were testing must be listed in this category.

Until these new drugs are released in the United States, your physician can only help with symptomatic treatment. There are many ways in which his or her skills may be used to assist in the bolstering of the Immune Response by prescribing medications that cannot be purchased "over the counter."

PAIN

Pain medication can be prescribed by your physician. You must remember, however, that drugs to relieve pain are a two-edged sword. Most medications for pain that are stronger than aspirin are addictive. That is the reason they can only be prescribed by a physician. The following are a few examples of drugs that MAY be ordered in your individual case.

Codeine is a mild narcotic. It is usually given in pill form and it relieves pain for about four hours. It has the disadvantage of often causing nausea and constipation. The drug is only addictive when taken for a longer period of time.

Meperidine hydrochloride (Demerol) is a synthetic drug which has an effect similar to morphine. When I was first starting medical practice, the drug was thought to be non-addictive. However, it was soon found to cause serious problems. It is an excellent drug for short term relief of pain.

Morphine is the historical classic narcotic medication. It relieves pain for approximately four hours and also promotes drowsiness and a sense of euphoria. The drug is a derivative of the opium plant, from which heroin, cocaine and codeine are also produced. Addiction and intestinal stasis are serious problems.

There is also an entire class of synthetic narcotics that may be prescribed by authorized physicians.

LOCAL ANESTHETICS

Your physician is able to order any of several local anesthetics (Please be reminded that none of the following cure Herpes, they merely relieve pain.):

For oral lesions, anesthetic troches may be prescribed.

For local skin lesions, topical anesthetic creams and lotions may be given. Be sure to discuss with your physician whether the medication contains hydrocortisone or does not. Many preparations do contain such steroids, and should not be used.

148

Aerosal sprays may be ordered to give temporary relief of pain. This particular aid is an excellent method of depositing the medication on the area where it can act, for the lesions do not need to be touched and there is less chance of autoinoculation.

Anesthetic ointments (Nupercainal) can give welcome relief. Remember the disadvantage of ointments on the lesions.

In extreme cases your physician may inject the area with local anesthetics. Such a procedure can give 4- to 6-hour relief. This cannot be used when the lesions are widespread because of the amount of anesthetic that must be injected may be harmful.

Melvin was dying of cancer when I first saw him. One of his serious complications was the Herpes in his mouth and throat. The medications and the disease had depressed his Immune Response to such an extent that the Herpes virus was able to gain a foothold and found no resistance. One of the things that tears at the heart of a doctor is to know that he can do little for a patient. This was the situation when Melvin greeted me. We had known each other for many years and loved each other dearly. He had called for me because a friend had said that I knew something about Herpes and he hoped that I could ease his problem.

I could do little. We prescribed Burrow's solution compresses to his lips, and xylocaine viscous topical anesthetics for the pain inside the mouth. This relieved the soreness so that he could eat a little. Eventually, the only relief available was Demerol and morphine. Most of the time that was spent with Melvin was simply to let him know that someone who cared for him was standing by. His death was a relief to him and to me in a way. A friend had no more suffering. But it was, and is, a monument to the frustration of this damnable disease, Herpes.

LOCAL TREATMENT

Ether or chloroform has been used to treat local lesions. It is thought that the chemical changes the outer shell of the virus so that replication cannot occur. This theory may or may not be true, but there does seem to be a definite drying of the lesions. I have used this technique with benefit.

Alcohol also has been used to help dry the lesions. If there are a limited number of vesicles or ulcers, this treatment is satisfactory. For patients having many lesions, it is too painful for my recommendation.

Idoxuridine (IDU). This drug has been used for several years. Its efficacy at this time is limited to Keratitis where it is of benefit. On many occasions, the medication has been put into ointment form but little effectiveness has been reported. It may be that, once again, the ointment hinders this drug.

It is possible that including the medication in some other medium may produce better results. Trials with a spray of IDU has been reported to be more beneficial.

Boric acid has also been reported to be of help. This can be applied in the ointment or in simple solution at home. Discuss this procedure with your physician.

Bea came to our clinic some months after the study had been completed. She had a recurrent Herpes bout. Six lesions were distributed over the labia. No ulcers were found in the vagina nor on the cervix. Because the medication which we were previously testing was no longer available, we treated the lesions with applications of ether.

Bea's lesions were gently washed with mild surgical

soap, and pat dried. When they were thoroughly clean, ether, the same chemical that is used in anesthesia, was applied with an applicator to each lesion. Because ether dries rapidly, this process was repeated three times. The patient received daily treatments in the clinic for a period of one week. Bea's lesions were dry, less inflamed, and nearly healed at the end of the course of treatment.

It was my impression that patients treated in this manner improved more rapidly than those who did not receive such care.

STRESS

Your physician can help most by wise and patient counsel in caring for you and your problems of stress. What is it in your particular life that makes you uptight? How can the tension be relieved? How can you understand your own problems? How can you best cope with those problems? These are prime targets in the boosting of your Immune Response, and a sensitive health counselor can be of enormous help to a Herpes sufferer.

Most of the time, a good relationship between physician or health counselor and the patient is all that is needed, but once in a while professionals in the field need to be called in consultation. Qualified psychologists or psychiatrists are important resources in those instances.

Laurie and Mark were devastated. In their late twenties, they had two children, fine jobs, and a beautiful new home. Their salaries were capable of handling all of their financial matters. Life seemed to be great until Herpes afflicted both. Where did it come from? Each accused the other of infidelity but each stated that their

151

fidelity was true. The problem was ripping the family apart.

Counseling brought out separately that each had had an affair several years in the past, before they were married. Both Laurie and Mark were afraid to tell the other about it. This guilt had grown until some trigger caused the virus to begin to replicate. Or perhaps an innocent exposure via a contaminated toilet seat, or health club shower or bench was enough to start a flare-up of the infection. Ultimately both had recurrences.

The counsellor was able to get both to recognize the beauty of their relationship and to look carefully at the frustration and futility of their destruction of the family by their continuing distrust. After an emotional struggle, love won. They rebuilt their trust relationship. And the Herpes episodes decreased and finally disappeared entirely.

I do not advise loading a patient's system with drugs to allay their tensions (Valium, Miltown etc.). These medications should only be used under the supervision of a highly trained professional. Valium particularly can become a substance upon which the body relies. Valium and alcoholic beverages do not go together at all. The result can be fatal. Please do not chastise your physician if you are not given a prescription for unlimited amounts of these very potent drugs. I'm hoping your doctor agrees with me that giving large amounts of medication—when strict supervision is impractical or impossible—is one of the worst types of medical care.

Ask your doctor to help with your personal problems. If she or he does not do this type of counseling, request a referral to someone who does. If you still do not get satisfactory help and personal answers to your questions, go to another doctor. All of the medical findings and the laboratory work that has been accumulated must be transferred to the new doctor for the new set of records. That is the law, and also the ethics of medical practice. If the practitioner refuses to send copies of all of your records to your new physician, contact the Medical Association or your attorney.

HERPES ENCEPHALITIS

One of the serious types of Herpes is that of involvement of the brain. A high rate of mortality accompanies this difficult diagnosis. Fortunately, a treatment is now available in which hope rests. The arabinoside family of drugs have been successful in reducing the rate of death from this problem. These drugs have side effects that give concern but, in life-threatening situations, they are used to advantage.

KERATITIS

The serious condition of ulcers of the cornea of the eye from the virus of Herpes has been treated successfully in a good percentage of cases using the drug, Idoxuridine. This is an efficient but not an ideal drug for the treatment. Some of the Herpes viruses are resistant. The same problem that exists whenever we try to treat deep infections with surface medication is present. When the deeper tissues of the cornea are infected the drug does not reach those areas. Recurrences of the flare-up are the result.

Adenine arabinoside also has been used in the treatment of this disease, and a similar success to that of IDU has been reported. The same problems which I have just described affect the results with this ointment-based medication.

There are not many choices that a physician has for drugs that are specific. Your doctor must rely, at this time, on but a few. He or she must also use the powers that they possess in the art of medicine, that ability to assist you in the care and prevention of the spread of this disease.

There are new aids on the way, however. These will be discussed in the next chapter.

Chapter 13

WHAT'S IN THE FUTURE FOR TREATMENT

There is a profusion of new medications undergoing testing. My hope is that some of these will be proven to be beneficial. All are withheld from general use because of the restrictions of the Food and Drug Administration. In the past, I have supported their efforts to control the proliferation of drugs in the United States. Certainly the prevention of the thalidomide problems is a great achievement, and for that action I am very grateful. However, the restrictions seem to result in withholding from the public, Herpes medications that research has proven valuable.

There are several classes of drugs that are being tested for use. These represent different approaches to combat the same problem. That problem is the Herpes virus itself. As you now know, the virus picks out nerve tissue in which to hide during the sometimes long latent period. This nerve tissue involves some of the most critical areas of the anatomy, ones that control muscle stimulation and sensation, and, of course, the brain. Medications must work in such a way that the nerves, and particularly the brain, are not altered nor damaged.

The various classes of the drugs being tested are:

The viricides. These chemicals kill the virus. Their action prevents the virus from carrying on its existence.

155

Virustatic drugs. The virus shell-altering drugs. This class works by so altering the covering of the virus that the replication ability is interrupted. Through this alteration of its mechanism of life, the ability to proliferate is lost.

The vaccines. This method of combating the virus is to develop a vaccine that will boost the residual antibody level in the system so that the virus cannot be effective.

Immunopotentiators. This new type of attack on disease is fascinating because it does nothing at all to the virus—but it boosts the Immune Response so that the body heals itself. The virus of Herpes remains as it has been, drowsing in the nerve tissue of the trigeminal nerve or the cauda equina.

I shall review each of these classes and discuss a few of the new drugs that are representative of each.

VIRICIDES

Idoxuridine (IDU)

This chemical has been under study since 1961. It is now effective in treating keratitis in a majority of cases. The problem with this local treatment was discussed in the last chapter.

Arabinosides

These drugs also were discussed under the heading of already authorized medications. Further work is being done to put these into acceptable formulas that will be of benefit to the sufferers of genital Herpes.

Acyclovir

Acyclovir has been authorized for use in humans in rare instances. Tests at Johns Hopkins School of Medicine seem to show that 20 patients given the drug did not develop Herpes lesions following bone marrow transplant. These sores are a common aftermath of such surgical procedures.

Animal studies show this drug to have antiviral capacities much greater than vidarabine or idoxuridine. However, testing in humans has a long way to go before toxicity studies have been completed. Only a relatively few patients have been given the drug to this date and these only in rather bizarre instances. The medication is given intravenously every eight hours for five days. Hospitalization is required.

Currently there is in the national press a great amount of publicity about its miraculous effects. Though the drug has not been completely tested, and the new reports are premature, and more in the nature of sensational news than in the reports of large scale studies, I believe that it has great promise. It will probably be more available within a few years.

VACCINES

BCG

Attention has been pointed toward BCG vaccine, which is derived from a bacillus related to the bacteria which causes tuberculosis. It is given after a Herpes infection or a recurrence in order to lessen symptoms and frequency. Dr. Lawerence Corey of the University of Washington, School of Medicine, reported to the American Society for Microbiology on a double-blind study. He came to the conclusion that the vaccine did not have a great value in the prevention of Herpes. His reports show that there may be a slight shortening of the duration of the symptoms.

Vaccine from Germany

One program from Germany involved a vaccine which required hundreds of injections. It received some praise in the early 70s. Today there is little that is heard of the regimen.

Vaccine from the United States

Several programs for testing viral vaccines are under way in the United States. Merck, Sharp and Dohme Research Laboratories are apparently testing vaccines at this time, but word of the results has not been reported widely.

IMMUNOPOTENTIATORS

Immunopotentiating drugs work in a most interesting manner. They do not seem to have much effect upon the virus itself but act to enhance our own Immune Response. Each of the two drugs which I shall discuss in this chapter is entirely different but the results of the action of each is similar.

Interferon

This drug may be of great importance in the future. It is a blood factor derivative and has the property of interfering with replication in a wide variety of DNA and RNA viruses.

Recently the importance of Interferon as an immune modulator has been recognized. Natural killer cell activity and macrophage actions can be enhanced by this chemical. The T-lymphocyte activity may also be increased.

There are problems with the drug. For one thing the drug is hard to get and very expensive. Most of the human leukocyte interferon used for clinical testing throughout the world comes from the one laboratory of Dr. Kari Cantell in Helsinki, Finland.

At present the drug is highly experimental, and very few projects are able to be carried out. It is tremen-

158

dously expensive and requires hospitalization for administration of the medication.

Much further study needs to be done before the drug will have general use. Determination of optimum dosage programs for Prophylaxis with patients must be calculated. Treatment of patients at high risk, those having cancer and Herpes zoster infections, kidney transplant recipients with cytomegalovirus infections, and patients with recurrent Herpes keratitis should be given priority.

The most comprehensive studies of the role of interferon in the treatment of virus infections have been carried out with patients who have a serious medical problem and then also become infected with Herpes zoster (shingles). The Immune Response in these patients is already severely depressed and the additional infection is a serious threat. Patients who were treated very early in the course of the disease with high doses of the medication showed a significant decrease of new vesicle formation, less immediate pain, and diminished lingering neuritis after the lesions had healed.

Herpes simplex labialis is also benefited when interferon is given for five days before surgery on the trigeminal nerve. Both the presence of the virus and the severity of the lip lesions were reduced, following the surgery.

Herpes simplex keratitis can be treated with vidarabine and idoxuridine. These compounds, though effective in helping to heal the lesions, do not prevent recurrences with corneal damage. Interferon, accompanied by debridement, the surgical procedure of clearing away of any damaged eye tissue, has been reported to accelerate healing.

Great help in many fields of medical care is anticipated for interferon, but until the problems of availability and cost are solved, probably through discovering a process for artificial synthesis, its use will not become

159

general. Perhaps these problems will be conquered within ten years.

THE EXPERIMENTAL MEDICATION

The drugs which I have described above have been utilized in limited studies. The medication, which we were testing at California State University, Fullerton, has been used widely and is authorized for use in 51 nations. Literally millions of doses of the medication have been given. The United States is one of the few nations in the world that does not allow its use.

It is impossible for me to write a comprehensive book on Herpes without mentioning the drug with which we worked. However, so much pressure has been brought to bear that I must apologize to you for not being allowed even to mention its name or the name of the small company that manufactures the compound in the United States. That company requests this because mention of the name might jeopardize the possible approval of the drug. The medication has not been approved by the FDA for use except under an experimental classification.

Even though I have been criticized by some for spending too much space in a discussion of the drug, this area is where much of my experience exists. My reference to this experimental drug is not to demean any of the other fine medications, for undoubtedly it is from these substances the solutions to Herpes will probably arise. The reason I elaborate upon the experimental drug is to describe some of the details of our program and to relate a few of the observations. When a patient came to the University Clinic with possible Herpes, he or she was interviewed to determine any significant history of past diseases, surgery, or medications. We were particularly interested in antibiotics and birth control pills or other hormones that the patient was taking at the time.

The patient was then examined physically. Blood tests were drawn and tests of the sores were made. Pap tests were taken to look for the giant multinuclear cells which are typical of Herpes. Those would also alert us to cancer if it were present. Virus cultures were taken from the moisture in the bottom of the lesions. Tests for gonorrhea and syphilis were carried out in order to rule out those diseases and the confusion that they might cause.

I photographed the lesions of each patient so that a chronological comparison could be made of the progress of each person's infection. This technique eliminated guesswork. And also provided a rare set of pictures of the disease.

We examined the patients every other day for two weeks and took further tests. As we were most interested in the liver function of the patients, studies were performed. Our interest in this portion of the problem related to the drug which we were testing, for the drug is a purine derivative and there is a potential that the medication might act adversely in someone with liver or kidney problems. Purines are chemicals which have uric acid as an end product. (Uric acid is found in the body in high concentration in cases of gout.) We found minimal evidence of this complication.

Because of the legal intricacies requiring parental consent, minors were eliminated from the study. Eighteen years is the age of majority in California.

We also eliminated pregnant women from the research for we felt that an outpatient clinic could not handle the potential problems that such care might bring. I regretted having to make such a decision because care of pregnancy has long been my special interest and joy. In California, the legal complications of such care are extreme.

When a patient was accepted into the program, he or she was given a supply of pills which was sufficient only for 48 hours. Giving so few pills was a ruse, but there was a genuine reason. It was important for the patient to return for observation of what was occurring. Each one was examined before receiving further medication. At each visit the lesions were observed, a chance for the patient to ask questions was given, the progress of the sores was photographed, and finally a new supply of pills were prescribed. Questions about progress were asked by me or by Mrs. Helen Lagerquist, R.N., the nurse who was my principal associate in the research program.

Medications were handled in a disciplined manner by only two pharmacists, Don Boals and Bert Harris. They were the only persons who dispensed the medication to the patients. None of the remainder of us who were on the team touched the medicine. All laboratory specimens were handled strictly by three technologists, Hilda Lanman and Gina Radas, who worked under Supervisor Carol Morrow. They were the only ones who completed the blood chemistry tests and handled the virus specimens. Some of these latter specimens were transferred to Dr. Jack Bradshaw's laboratory for testing of the PHA levels, which reflect the Immune Response of the patient.

The clinical staff was also strictly limited and specially trained. I personally examined each patient at each visit. One backup physician, gynecologist Dr. Richard Hayden, assisted. The nursing staff, under the direction of Arlene Myers, consisted of Helen Lagerquist and her backup, Dorothy Uno. The staff was limited in number in order to ascertain responsibility and training. The remainder of the Clinic staff and the entire University was intensely interested in the project, and Mrs. Lagerquist and I gave many lectures on the subject of Herpes.

As I have stated, anecdotes do not reflect the true results of a study, but a double-blind research program can be given more credence. I shall report further on the cold statistics, for we were amazed by the results, but first let me illustrate some of the cases which I observed.

I have reported the activities of Ted, the water skier, many times. Perhaps some of you have gotten to know him through the several chapters. Because Ted was a graduate student at the University and interested in the subject, we kept in touch for several years. He regularly came into my office for a chat and so I could examine his lips.

After the results of the double-blind program were completed and released to us, we found Ted was one of the subjects that had received the active medication. He also kept up his same lifestyle of going to the Colorado River water skiing. After the one week of medication which was given during the test, he had no more fever blisters for eleven months. This was with no further medication. Ted subsequently re-entered the study and, on the second trial, received the placebo. His fever blisters continued unabated.

Paula enjoyed oral sex. She arrived at the clinic three days after an evening with her boyfriend. The vulva was covered with lesions. I counted about twenty. The sores were red, moist, and deeply cratered. They covered the mons, circled the clitoris, and spread out onto the swollen labia. The opening to the vagina was covered with the ulcers. She was in agony.

Paula was admitted to the study and started on the test medication. Because she was in so much pain we requested that she return the following day.

Paula strode into the clinic 24 hours later for her appointment. Her lesions had lost most of the redness and much of the moisture. The swelling of the labia was much less. She was having no pain.

On subsequent visits, Paula was found to have no new sores. The old ones cleared quickly. She reported that she had no further pain. She was astonished and joyful.

Paula was one of the group who received the test drug.

Joan also was seen following oral sex. The lesions were scattered over the labia and the mons. Painful and red, they caused her much discomfort. She was started on the medication after the preliminary work-up. Joan's lesions subsided in eleven days and the pain lessened only gradually shortly before the last day.

When the results were made available to us, it was found that Joan had received the placebo.

Dennis had recurrent Herpes. There were scars of previous infections along the shaft of the penis and a shiny crusted area in the midshaft on the dorsal surface and the side. There were three small ulcers on the scrotum.

Dennis was admitted to the study. For three days new lesions were evident and small vesicles were seen. There were enlarged lymph nodes in both groin areas.

Following the three-day period, no new lesions were observed. There was no pain in the area. The inflammation disappeared and the lesions had dry crusts. No change in the lymph node enlargement was noted. Dennis, too, proved in retrospect to have taken the active medication. His own report of the discomfort was based on many experiences with bouts of the disease. He stated that this episode was far less painful than any previous one.

* * *

Sonia had a fever blister and sores in her mouth. She loved the sun and reinforced her California tan whenever possible. She told me that repeatedly she would develop cold sores which often extended into the inner surfaces of her lips. When I saw her, this type of episode was evident. A large and confluent fever blister spilled over into her mouth from her lower lip. There were many canker sores.

She was admitted to the study and was given the medication which was later proven to be the active drug. The lip lesions dried in four days and two days later her mouth was clear.

Thelma had only a few Herpes sores. They were only slightly painful. Located in the folds of the inner part of the vagina, they were difficult to visualize. When I was able to observe the lesions adequately, it was obvious that the craters were that of Herpes. The culture and the microscopic study for giant multinuclear cells confirmed the clinical suspicion.

Thelma was also started on the active drug and the lesions disappeared in three days.

In Chapter 2, I wrote about Debbie. She was carried into our clinic by her husband, unable to walk because of the serious sores in the vagina. She also had keratitis and lesions on her shoulders, back, breasts, knees, and legs. There were many lesions in her mouth. Debbie had Behcet's Syndrome.

She and her husband pleaded with us to admit her to the study and we complied. The virus cultures were positive in all the areas mentioned. She was started on the test drug.

When Debbie returned the next day, there was a marked change in her condition. The redness had progressed from scarlet to maroon and there was much less inflammation surrounding the 1- by 2-inch vaginal ulcers. The pain was less. She was able to walk.

The PHA test (the blood chemistry test which indicates the body's resistance) was markedly low.

On the third day, Debbie walked happily into the clinic. Her eye was not red. The lesions on the shoulder, breast, knees, and shins were not visible and the massive ulcers in the vagina were not inflamed. We could not believe it when she stated that there was no pain. The photographs reveal a different woman from the one who first sought our counsel.

I am sorry to say that Debbie was lost to the study because of an unrelated problem which required hospitalization.

All I can report is that in three days, Debbie made enormous improvement. I cannot feel that the result was that of a placebo.

These case histories bear out what I have observed. But they are just individual results. One good shot does not a golfer make, nor does one case history (or three or ten) a worthwhile drug prove.

Let us look at but two of the many cold statistics of the study: the incidence of new lesion development after the test drug has been started and the overall cure rate of the course of treatment for one episode.

There were no new lesions formed in any patient who was taking the medication after the third day of the study. In my opinion this is a very significant finding, for new lesions were still being formed after ten days in some of the patients who were taking the placebo.

The following graph helps illustrate. The percentage of patients showing new vesicle formation is on the verticle bar to the left. The number of days of treatment is shown in the horizontal bar. The dotted line for the test drug ends at the third day. Those patients treated with the placebo, the solid line, continues.

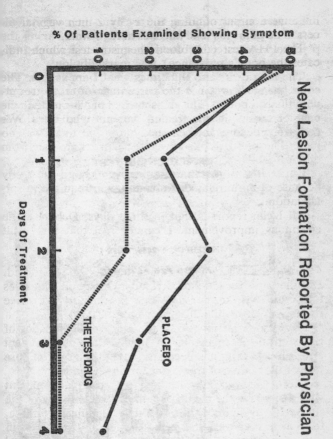

% Of Patients Examined Showing Symptom

New Lesion Formation Reported By Physician

Days Of Treatment

THE TEST DRUG

PLACEBO

We found that there were many other symptoms show-ing improvement: pain, itching, and lymph node size. However, the statistic which I most wish to bring to your attention is the final one, that of the individual episode cure rate. We found that those patients taking the test drug were cured of their Herpes bout in nearly 60% of the cases at the end of one week. Those taking the placebo were cured, by the same criteria, in about 14% of the cases.

The next chart also illustrates what I am saying. The solid bar at the right is the percentage of those treated with the compound. The crosshatched bar shows the per-cent of those placebo-treated patients who were over their Herpes sores in one week.

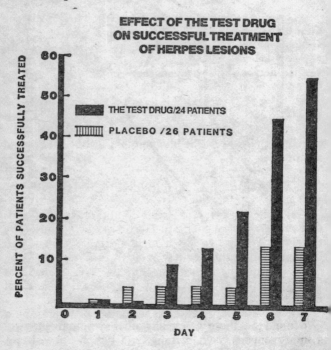

EFFECT OF THE TEST DRUG
ON SUCCESSFUL TREATMENT
OF HERPES LESIONS

PERCENT OF PATIENTS SUCCESSFULLY TREATED

■ THE TEST DRUG/24 PATIENTS
▨ PLACEBO /26 PATIENTS

DAY

When I speak about the test compound, I am usually asked the excellent question, "What are the side effects?"

My experience is based on our study. We observed side effects during the research program. But there were more side effects reported among the patients taking the placebo than among the drug-treated group. The following chart lists all of the side effects complained about by the patients. Several complaints each came from six of the patients studied.

SIDE EFFECTS

	The Test Drug	Placebo
Gastrointestinal	5	5
Genitourinary	4	3
Musculoskeletal	7	4
Central nervous system (headache)	3	8
Others	2	2
TOTAL	**21**	**22**

All of the side effects encountered in our study were minor ones.

TREATMENT OF HERPES ENCEPHALITIS

As I stated in Chapter 2, this condition is a very serious but rare complication of Herpes. Usually caused by the Type 1 virus, it has a high mortality and a high incidence of residual effects in survivors.

Treatment has so far been limited to arabiniside or idoxuridine. Most reports show that those drugs are not ideal.

The same experimental compound was studied by a group of French neurologists. The drug is authorized in France, Germany, Italy, Japan, and Spain, among the technical nations of the world.

A report appearing in the *Review of Neurology*

(Paris), 1979, discussed seven cases which were confirmed or probable acute necrotizing (disintegrating) Herpes encephalitis. Six of the seven cases were treated with the medication.

Four of the six patients with encephalitis recovered from the previously 80% fatal disease.

One case history which was cited in the report illustrates the course.

Helene was 23 years of age and was hospitalized for acute psychosis. Her symptoms had started fifteen days before admission. She had had fever and an upper respiratory infection. Four days later she was disoriented and amnesic. She even forgot to go to an examination at the University. A week passed and behaviorial disorders began. She made motiveless cries, screams, and was agitated. She tried to bite objects. Hallucinations began and she was hospitalized. Within a few days language disorders started, and shortly afterward she suffered a grand mal seizure, which is a convulsion or fit.

Many tests and electroencephalograms were performed. These tests culminated in the diagnosis of encephalitis. Many neurological signs persisted. The patient was started on the test drug after another EEG. The drug was given for a period of fifteen days. Following treatment, during the fifth week a surprising and rapid improvement in the clinical state was observed with almost total disappearance of the disorders. Six weeks later Helene returned to the University with a normal EEG.

In spite of the fact that there is abundant evidence of the benefit of the drug and there have been almost no side effects reported in our study and in those of many other studies from the United States and around the

170

world, the Food and Drug Administration has held back this medication from general use.

Previously I wrote of several diseases that are similar to Herpes. The treatment of those diseases is important also. The next chapter covers that subject.

Chapter 14

ANTICIPATED TREATMENTS FOR SIMILAR DISEASES

Diseases caused by similar viruses to that of Herpes often have similar characteristics. The discussion of these problems can be found in Chapter 7. Therapies for these conditions are often as elusive as the treatment for Herpes itself. Let us look again at some of these diseases and new drugs that are on the way.

HERPES ZOSTER

Shingles is often calamitous in older age persons. As with the Herpes simplex virus it is believed that 100% of the population harbor the varicella-zoster virus. The exquisitely painful lesions which occur in this disease may be permanent because of scarring of the extremely delicate and sensitive nerve endings.

Because of the dire consequences, it is imperative that a treatment for the disease be found.

Herpes zoster is also a serious complication in immunosuppressed persons, people whose Immune Response is depleted. Patients undergoing therapy for cancer are at higher risk of contracting shingles. People with Hodgkins Disease and those having bone marrow transplants are particularly susceptible. For these persons, too, finding a cure is vital.

THE EXPERIMENTAL DRUG

In an article in the *Journal of the American Medica[l] Association,* of July 1981, famed Dr. Albert B. Sabin developer of the polio vaccine, reports that a vaccin[e] for Herpes zoster has been developed by Dr. Takahash[i] and his group in Japan. The therapy has undergon[e] extensive testing there. Dr. Sabin recomends that ef forts to duplicate the excellent results of the Japanes[e] investigators should be stepped up.

Independent work here in the United States must b[e] done before the Food and Drug Administration will b[e] satisfied and will authorize the use of any program.

Because of very successful reports from outside o[f] the United States, I have been interested in the use of th[e] test drug in several cases. The results have been amaz ing.

Warren was retired. He had worked hard all his lon[g] life in service to humankind. He still kept busy. Be cause I was a friend, he called when a rash broke ou[t] on his right side. I found a row of blisters about tw[o] inches wide, clustered from the center of the chest. Th[e] inexact line extended under the arm and across th[e] back to the spinal column. There were six groups o[f] vesicles. His pain was severe.

I explained that there was no treatment available i[n] the United States. I also stated that the drug we ha[d] been testing was available in Mexico but that I coul[d] not legally recommend it. He procured the medicatio[n] himself.

After two days of therapy, the lesions were painless dry, and noninflamed.

* * *

Clara was the mother of one of my associates. On the plane to a Hawaiian vacation, she began to experience pain in the left side of her neck, scalp, and forehead. By the time they reached the hotel, lesions of Herpes zoster were evident.

My colleague made arrangements for some medication to be flown to the Islands.

Though therapy was not started as soon as desirable, the pain disappeared within two days and the lesions dried much faster than would be expected. One of the lesions was near the left eye, but no infection developed on the cornea.

My wife, Jean, had abdominal surgery. On the seventh post operative day, after she was home and doing very well, she began to complain of severe pain in the right side of the abdomen. The problem was very localized to an area four inches lateral to the incision. When I came home from the office, there were lesions typical of Herpes zoster in an oval cluster the size of a silver dollar. Jean, who is a stoic, said the pain was much worse than the surgical incision.

She began on therapy at suppertime.

Jean called me at my office at 10 o'clock the next morning and stated, "Dear, I have no pain."

The lesions progressed not at all from that point. They lost the fiery red color and dried up over the next few days. No further clusters broke out. There was no residual neuritis, the scourge of shingles.

These case histories are anecdotal. However, from my observations and from the many reports from other countries, I attach more significance to the results than to that of a placebo. There has not been a single failure among the persons which I have observed. (Inciden-

175

tally, medication taken by these patients was procure
by them outside of the United States.)

INFECTIOUS MONONUCLEOSIS

Though infectious mononucleosis is apparentl
caused by a Herpes-like virus, little progress has bee
made toward specific treatment of this disease of youn
people.

Prevention is best, and the same techniques which
advised for prevention of Herpes are worthwhile in thi
disease. Remember that prevention is hard work an
often means a change of lifestyle. (Please refer to Chap
ter 10 for details of prevention techniques.)

Other therapy for mono is symptomatic. Bed rest
important. I advise students, except in rare instances, t
continue to attend classes. They are not allowed to par
ticipate in any sports and are instructed to be lyin
down for at least one hour every afternoon. They ca
study then, but studying in bed is not good for th
concentrative abilities. At least eight hours of sleep i
important.

No athletics are allowed during the course of the dis
ease for two prime reasons. Exhaustion prolongs th
length of time before recovery, and the spleen, which i
an organ in the upper part of the abdomen, may b
enlarged ten times its usual fist-like size. The spleen ca
easily be damaged at such a time by trauma. The resu
can be fatal, and at a minimum, necessitates abdomina
surgery.

As fever is a problem, aspirin is advisable and eve
cooling baths and blankets which are moistened, wrun
out of cool water, and placed upon the patient may b
needed. The blankets are changed frenquently until th
cooling effect has been accomplished. Antibiotics do n
good in mononucleosis, but are often important in com

batting a secondary infection. Corticosteroids, though nonspecific, are sometimes used to great benefit.

POLIOMYELITIS

Dr. Sabin's recent article, to which I previously referred, comments not only on the three types of polioviruses but also on the nineteen other enteroviruses which can occasionally cause paralysis. New vaccines need to be developed for the other viruses. He stressed again that polio still occurs in many parts of the world and, through the wonders of modern travel, can be introduced into any community at any time. It is imperative for all children to be vaccinated.

CYTOMEGALIC INCLUSION DISEASE

This disease is caused by the cytomegalovirus and is a frequent problem in humans and in animals such as monkeys and rodents. Over 25 years have gone by since these viruses were isolated and research is continuing into the myriad effects that occur.

Since the early 1970s, this virus has come to be felt to play a very significant part in the success or failure of organ transplantation procedures. In addition, there is recognition that infants who are congenitally infected but apparently asymptomatic at birth may, in later years, show severe hearing defects and possibly a lowered mental ability.

This disease, similar to that of the Herpes simplex viruses, may be transmitted through sexual contact. It has been added to the general list of venereally transmitted entities.

When a newborn arrives into the world, the secretions of the cervix and the vagina come into intimate contact with it. Presence of the virus in those secretions has been detected in many studies since it was first reported by Japanese investigators in 1970. There appears to be little organ selectivity with this disease as there is with the Herpes virus which seems to attack the areas of nerve distribution. Because of the wide possibilities of contact at birth, there are many areas of the body that may be involved. The liver is not infrequently infected. Hepatitis is the result. Pneumonia occasionally occurs. The virus is sometimes found in the intestinal tract of the newborn. Eye and ear infections have been felt to result from this problem.

The cytomegalovirus has been found in blood transfusions and such an exposure seems to have resulted in a mononucleosis-like problem in the recipient.

In renal organ transplant patients the picture is most often that of fever, muscle aches and arthralgias, a lowering of the white blood count, poor liver function, and lung involvement. These events tend to occur within a few months of the time of the surgical procedure.

Research is taking a most interesting direction in the last few years and the answers are not nearly complete, but studies on the relationship of the pancreas and cytomegalovirus is being looked at. There is some indication that the area of the organs that have to do with insulin production and the disease of diabetes may be involved. It is hoped that this virus may be considered in future research that is directed toward the possible viral cause of juvenile diabetes.

The frequency of the disease is quite common and there is a good probability that few persons escape the problem during their lifetime. However, the usual course of events is that there are few symptoms and the diagnosis is made by a specific antibody response. The disease is more significant in the newborn and in the world approximately 1 percent of babies are born with the condition.

The diagnosis of the disease is best made by isolation of the virus through culture. Electron microscopy is also useful but the virus is difficult to distinguish from other similar viruses. In addition, there are a number of blood tests that are becoming more specific in solidifying the diagnosis.

Like other virus diseases, there are new treatments that seem to show promise of solving many of the problems of this puzzler.

VACCINE

Vaccines are being tested and give hope of being effective. They do engender concern on the part of some researchers but the work is becoming more and more developed. In the human subjects that were tested antibodies against the virus were developed. These chemical evidences of the virus show that the body's defenses were stimulated by the vaccine. We shall undoubtedly hear more of this research in the future.

ANTIVIRALS

Some of the antivirals which are active against the Herpes virus are being tested in the control of the cytomegalovirus, also. The result in some of the laboratory studies have been promising but the clinical trials have been reported to lack the hoped for beneficial effect. Some of the drugs that have been tested are idoxuridine and the arabinoside family.

ACYCLOVIR

Acyclovir has been tested and some beneficial effect has been reported, but it has not been quite as strong as the recent reports relative to Herpes. The national press did publish information about the benefit of the drug in organ transplant recipients a few months ago.

INTERFERON

There has been much interest in this compound for the treatment and prevention of the disease. The results

179

of the treatment apparently have not been as desirable as at first thought but the prevention, particularly in cases involving organ transplants, has been more successful.

As with the Herpes there are many problems in the testing and authorization of an effective treatment. We will hear more of the results in the future but, in the meantime, we must be thankful for our own immune system that wards off so many of the virus infections.

Chapter 15

WHAT IF I'M PREGNANT?

Jane, this chapter is written especially for you. A long time has passed since I wrote the Foreword and mentioned that you attended one of my lectures. You left crying, for you had Herpes and were pregnant. You wanted to have your baby by Natural Childbirth. I had said that probably a Caesarean Section delivery was indicated. You left the lecture room in tears and I couldn't get to you.

WHY THE CONCERN?

Jane, the reason for concern of delivery through the birth canal in the presence of Herpes lesions is real and very serious. Serious for your newborn infant. I wish I did not have to write to you of this, but it is necessary so that you will have all the facts upon which to base your opinions and actions. If a mother has positive cultures of Herpes virus at the time of delivery, there is a 40–60% chance of the baby becoming infected. Of babies so infected, 50% will develop a generalized infection with Herpes virus disease. Brain damage or death is the expected result. Every preventive measure possible must be utilized to avoid this tragedy.

The chances are good that as term approaches your Herpes lesions will not be active and there will be no virus shedding. Your doctor will take cultures from the vagina and cervix to determine this. If no virus is found, natural delivery may be encouraged.

There are ways in which you can help, too, to eliminate triggers which may cause flare-ups. I have been discussing these for many pages but for a short review, a few of those are:

PREVENTION

CLEANLINESS

Cleanliness implies the hard work of washing hands, body, clothes, and linens.

Washing the vulva and the perineum, and urinating before and after sex are also very important.

SEX

I would strongly recommend abstaining from sex completely for the last three months before your due date in order to eliminate one more trigger that might initiate an episode of Herpes.

REST

Rest is important. It gives your body a time of freedom from strains and physical exertion so that your defenses can be replenished. Fatigue is a trigger that should be avoided.

I know it is hard to get comfortable as term approaches. The best preparation begins way back when you are first pregnant. I hope that you have been continuing your desire for Natural Childbirth and working hard with the techniques of relaxation, for it is a great advantage and adventure to your new baby and you.

NATURAL CHILDBIRTH IN PREGNANT HERPES PATIENTS

The several techniques of Natural Childbirth will help you in many ways: to maintain good muscle support, to help control your muscles so you can voluntarily relax your body, to assist in knowledge of what is happening to you, and reducing and controlling stress.

Preparation for childbirth by whatever technique you choose is important because of the close relationship that is engendered between patient and doctor. It is a two-way avenue of caring, trust, and confidence.

You must have faith in your obstetrician—and the person guiding your obstetrical care should have faith in you.

Your guide has had special training and has knowledge and experience that you have not had, continuous updating in the field of obstetrics and gynecology, and the main experience of delivering babies. After 4,000 deliveries, I was vastly more knowledgeable than after ten or even one hundred.

And so, Jane, one of the first things that I hope for you is that you are able to find an obstetrician in whom you have confidence and to whom you can talk, a doctor who will relate to you as a person and not as a medical specimen. The doctors who are just beginning practice today, Jane, have superb training. It is broadbased and usually finishes with some particular special interest area. You have a special problem, and I hope that you have freedom of discussion with your obstetrician.

Acting upon your doctor's advice—taking it—is your responsibility, but be certain you understand what is recommended before you accept that counsel—or reject it.

Jane, the joy of childbirth is threefold: mother's, father's and baby's. As a doctor I thrill each time it happens, but my position is that of a coach, an outsider. The doctor must have the responsibility and your cooperation, too, to act as a coach and change the plays, if the situation of your life or the baby's warrants.

Your most serious concern, now that delivery time is near, may be Caesarean Section. Your doctor must have the right to make that recommendation and you must give it your utmost consideration. The decision is ultimately yours, but you must not be more cavalier in rejecting the advice than your physician should be in giving it.

We are now concerned with the delivery of your baby in a manner which will add most to the infant's strength and its ability to resist infection by the Herpes virus—to add in every way possible to the Immune Response. The more natural a birth can be, the greater is the mother's Immune Response—and consequently she transfers a greater Immune Response to the infant.

I delivered more than 2,500 babies by Natural Childbirth. The difference in my life from the previous 1,500 was like night and day. For one thing, having to resuscitate infants who were zonked because their mothers were over-narcotized or overanesthetized is a stress-producing business. It's scary for me to have to be exceedingly gentle and accomplish the traumatic procedure of placing a tube in a tiny infant's windpipe. And before I became interested in Natural Childbirth, I had to, many times.

After I had delivered the first 1,500 babies, I met Dr. Sir Lance Townsend, heard his lectures, and we became friends. He is an Australian obstetrician and gynecologist, and now the Dean of the University of Melbourne, School of Medicine. A world authority in his field, he was the first Australian physician to be knighted by the Queen of the British Empire. He changed my entire medical practice and even my outlook on life. He taught me about Natural Childbirth.

184

The last 2,500 babies were delivered without the necessity of resuscitation of more than a dozen infants, and some of those were births in which I was called by the nurses to assist another physician in handling a case.

One case story is notable. It happened the night before I left private practice in order to join the faculty of the University. A patient of mine was in labor and it seemed slow. I knew from previous deliveries that suddenly this young lady could dilate and deliver so I had better be near. My patient and her husband were chatting and she was fine.

About 5 AM I was in the nurses' station drinking a cup of coffee that had started brewing at 11 PM. Suddenly we heard a baby crying. Such an event in a labor room galvanizes everyone like an electric shock. We dashed into the labor suite to find the faint cry. It was coming from under the blankets of another doctor's patient. The mother was still sound asleep. She was out cold from the medication that had been ordered.

How long had that infant been without rigorous respiration or assistance is something no one can ever tell. The baby seemed to be OK but we will never know the number of brain cells that may have been damaged during those moments. Such an event can result in a lower Immune Response and could cause an infant to be more susceptible to contracting its mother's Herpes.

Most hospitals frown on such large amounts of medication, and trained anesthesiologists are usually called to assist at delivery. For this we can be exceedingly grateful. However, some patients are hypersensitive to drugs and such an event can still happen. Today, fetal monitors tell us of the situation of the heart of the infant so we are much more sure, but a better way is needing less medication for relaxation.

In contrast, it was the choice of the vast majority of my patients to have little or no predelivery narcotics.

They had but to ask and a small dosage would be pro vided. But most didn't ask, for they eagerly awaited the excitement of being a part of bringing a new life into the world.

Jane, if it is the advice of your obstetrician that delivery in the normal manner is all right, one bit of routine may be varied from that of your friends' deliveries. For them the fetal monitor electrodes may have been placed against the baby's head as the cervix began to dilate. Because of the possibility of the monitors transferring Herpes to the infant, these devices are not recommended in usual deliveries when there is a history of mother or father having Herpes lesions. Your pediatrician and obstetrician should consult together and advise on their use.

Most of the babies delivered by Natural Childbirth techniques arrive into the world screaming joyously for something to eat. These lusty bellows begin the instant most are born. It is exciting to be a part of this ever recurring series of miracles. It is a joy for mother and father—and for the one who is assisting in the delivery. Observing such a miracle as birth is an excitement that for me is even greater today than it was when I first began to practice medicine many years ago.

Jane, the more you know about delivery and how to help through relaxation and training, the less anesthetic you will require. Your baby will have a stronger start, and with a history of Herpes, every possible boost to the infant should be given.

Even in the event of a Caesarean Section, many of the techniques advocated in Natural Childbirth can be utilized. This should be discussed with your physician.

DIET

Your diet is important. Remember Chapter 10 and the section on foods to eat and ones to avoid. Consult our obstetrician about having a diet not only rich in the usual vitamins and minerals but also in vitamin C, and ysine. Avoid argenine. I have seen no articles on the relation between diet and Herpes and pregnancy, but I can think of no reason to not follow such a program.

SMOKING

Smoking has ill effects, Jane, from many areas. There is a general debility and a smaller average size of the infants that is noted by many authors who compare babies of mothers who smoke with those of mothers who do not smoke.

In addition, my concern about Herpes and smoking holds true with women who are pregnant as well as those who are not.

My advice: don't smoke.

HOW DO I KNOW IF THERE'S TROUBLE?

Determinations of the risk will be made by your doctor every few days prior to delivery. Cultures of the vaginal or cervical sores or the lesions of the vulva may be taken. This is simple to do as only some of the moisture will be taken by swabbings with a cotton applicator. Culture is the most accurate way of determining virus shedding.

Another technique that will probably be used for a more rapid evaluation is to take Pap tests and look for the giant multinuclear cells which I have previously described.

CAESAREAN SECTION

Jane, you were concerned when I talked about Caesarean Section. It is the foremost preventive measure at

this time, and will probably be advised if there is evidence of active Herpes.

A "C. Section" is a major surgical procedure which
has been performed hundreds of thousands of times and
is quite safe. You must understand when I state this
that there is risk with any kind of surgery. There is also
risk with having a baby even without the complication
of Herpes or any other infection. The risk of Caesarean
Section is not much different from that.

As we are discussing Herpes, the usual considera-
tions in thinking about a Caesarean are not uppermost.
The relation of the size or position of the infant to the
size of the mother's pelvis is not the prime criterion.
The decision rests on the facts of the maturity of the
infant (how close the baby is to full term), the Herpes
infection itself, and the rupture of the mother's membranes (whether or not the water has broken).

One of the problems with Herpes is that of prematurity. Your obstetrician may use several techniques to determine the baby's age and vigor so as to avoid the additional complication of a premature infant. These
methods of measuring will be discussed with you. It is
probable that you would be allowed to begin labor so
that as much time of growth as possible would be given.

The decision to operate will be made also on whether
or not the membranes have ruptured. It is felt that there
are defensive antibodies in the amniotic fluid (the water) that help to prevent the virus from infecting the
fetus before birth. These antibodies have been determined in several studies. However, if the membranes
have been ruptured for four hours or more, the virus
can extend into the uterus and the chance of infection
of the infant is greatly increased. If the membranes
have been ruptured for that length of time, Caesarean
Section to prevent Herpes of the infant is no longer
valid and probably would be avoided unless there was
some other obstetrical problem.

The surgical procedure of Caesarean Section involves cleansing the abdomen thoroughly, administering an anesthetic to the patient, and the use of sterile techniques by the operating team. The team consists of a surgeon, an assistant surgeon, an anesthesiologist (usually all are physicians), and two or more nurses. The presence of a pediatrician or other physician to care for the infant is customary and vital.

An incision is made in the abdomen of the mother, usually crossways at the upper level of the pubic hair or from the unbilicus to the pubis in the midline. The tissues beneath are also exposed and the large flat muscles of the abdomen are retracted to each side. The urinary bladder is just underneath these structures and has already been deflated by being drained with a catheter. The plastic-like tissue which lines the abdomen and covers the bladder is incised and retracted. The bladder is in this way removed from the operating field and out of danger of injury.

Beneath the bladder lies the lower portion of the uterus and the cervix. This muscle is very thin when pregnancy is near term. Usually there is no difficulty making a small incision that can be enlarged enough toward each side to allow the baby's head to be born. The shoulders and trunk are then delivered, usually without difficulty. The process from the time of the incision to the delivery of the infant may often be completed as quickly as 5 minutes.

The infant is turned upside down so that any fluid which has been in its mouth may be removed. In a few moments the unbilical cord is cut and tied. This is usually after the cord has stopped pulsating.

The placenta (afterbirth) is removed through the same incision. The uterus then contracts strongly and almost immediately shrinks from the size of a watermelon to the size of a cantaloupe.

Next the layers of tissue and muscle that have been

incised are reapproximated with suture and the abdominal incision is closed. The entire operation may be completed in 30 to 45 minutes.

If there are no complications, Jane, you as the patient, will be up and around your room the next day or even the same day.

Following the delivery, the pediatrician and the pediatric nurse will make sure the baby is breathing well by cleansing any mucous from its mouth and pharynx. Because of the possibility of Herpes, the baby may be placed in an isolation room, where the pediatrician will do a thorough examination. The infant's skin, mouth, eyes, heart, lungs, and other tissues will be examined to assess the condition. Blood studies and perhaps virus cultures will be taken.

The care of the infant is approximately the same whenever the mother has a history of Herpes even if the delivery is natural. Isolation is usual because many times skin lesions do not begin to appear until a week or more after delivery. It is absolutely imperative not to spread the infection from one infant to another in the hospital nursery. The same disastrous results can occur from the disease that is transmitted in this manner as that which is contracted during the birth process.

Jane, I believe you want to nurse your baby. This is fine whether you deliver in the natural way or even if Caesarean Section is done. Caution has to be advised, however, for there have been a few cases reported of Herpes virus being isolated from mother's milk. Herpes lesions may develop in the nipple area of the breasts. Maintain strict sterility of breast shields and pads. Wash the nipples gently but thoroughly before and after nursing. Remember to rinse completely as this removes the soap and also flushes down the drain any virus particles that may possibly be present. If you have any sores on your skin near the nipple, a shield or plastic cover is important. Immediately consult your pediatrician or obstetrician.

If you have active Herpes when your baby is born, your doctor and educational nurse will make a special situation for you. Much instruction should be given you on how to protect the baby from becoming infected. These rules must be strictly followed.

INFECTION CONTROL PROCEDURES

The following brief outline is presented to you so that some guidance will be available to you to think about. This partial list is divided into categories depending on the infectivity of the mother. Your obstetrician, pediatrician, or hospital undoubtedly has classifications that are much more extensive.

The three classes I shall discuss are:
1. Active lesions or active virus shedding
2. A past history of active Herpes
3. Active non-genital Herpes (herpes labialis)

CLASS 1:

Active lesions or active virus shedding

The mother, and as far as possible, other family members, should be educated regarding risks that Herpes may cause to the infant, both in the hospital and at home. It is imperative that the mother understands the why of the various protective measures so that she can insist on their being followed at home—by everyone. If the mother is known to have lesions, the education should be started well in advance of the delivery—whether a Caesarean Section is contemplated or not.

Sexual activity should be avoided in the last 3 months of pregnancy. For women who will not abstain,

191

condoms, jellies, foams, and thorough washing of the vulva before and after coitus is advised.

Remember to urinate before and after sexual activity. Drink enough liquid to make this part of the process possible.

Do not forget that oral-genital sex can also transmit the virus.

Infection Control

In the hospital an infected mother should have a private room. Sterile gowns and gloves should be used for examination of a mother with active Herpes by all who come into contact with contaminated areas or articles. This includes doctors, nurses, and attendants.

Perineal pads and dressings which cover the infected area must be handled by double bagging—placing the contaminated material in one fresh plastic bag and sealing it. That bag is then placed in another bag and again sealed.

The mother may handle and feed her baby under supervised conditions. She should be out of bed and seated in a chair and should wear a newly laundered gown and gloves. Thorough hand scrubbing is less sterile but may be utilized.

In the hospital, after the above has been completed, the baby is brought to her. She may view the baby at the nursery after thorough hand washing and a fresh gown. She may not under any circumstances enter the nursery.

Care for the baby

The baby should be kept in a special care, isolation unit.

Gown and glove precautions should be used by all who attend the infant—doctors, nurses, and aides.

Contaminated articles should be double bagged.

Infants should be examined frequently for Herpes.

192

(Usually the disease breaks out within 12 days of birth.)

Care at home

The mother's care should continue as close as possible to hospital care as long as she has active lesions. When those lesions heal, fresh gowning and thorough washing may be used.

The family must also learn to use strict techniques of thorough washing, donning gowns, and avoiding contact with the infant whenever possible.

As the infection does not usually break out in the hospital, any sores on the skin of the newborn should be reported to the physician in charge immediately.

CLASS 2:

A Past History of Active Herpes

A patient who does not have evidence of virus shedding and who has no evidence of active lesions can usually be delivered in the normal manner, through the birth canal.

The mother does not need to be isolated and sterile handling techniques do not usually have to be used.

The baby does not need to be isolated.

At home a continuing observation of the infant should be carried out, and the family should be alert to report any lesions to the pediatrician.

No special isolation techniques need be observed for mother or infant at home, in the absence of lesions in either mother or child.

CLASS 3:

A Patient With Active Non-genital Herpes

In the hospital, a mother who has active non-genital Herpes should be observed carefully. She can usually deliver normally. Hand washing and fresh gowns should be used to protect the infant.

A mother who has fever blisters should be masked when handling her newborn.

Babies of mothers who have non-genital lesions should be isolated after they have been taken to the mother. After that visit they must be regarded as having been exposed and are a potential hazard to other infants.

Well, Jane, I have finished this chapter. I wish it was over for you. But you still must be careful, for you have had Herpes. It is imperative that you watch for problems in the future.

Chapter 16

IS IT CANCER?

David, I'm thinking of you as I write this chapter. You, almost hysterically, pushed past my secretary and burst into my office at 5 PM several months ago. You worriedly explained that you had had sex with your fiancée while you had lesions of Herpes. As you came through the door you nearly screamed, "I just gave cancer to the girl I love!"

We had a long talk then, David, for you had just read a frightening article in a slick magazine which gave you that impression.

I wish I could say that your fiancée, and you, have no need to worry but I cannot. My only statement is that there is a possibility of cancer but it is remote. There are things that can be accomplished to prevent that cancer from being neglected, for that is the kind to fear.

Let's discuss the topic of Herpes and cancer under four parts, David, and perhaps some of your concerns will be eased, others may be clarified, and still others will give your fiancée and you some definite precautions upon which you can concentrate your activities.

1. You cannot transmit cancer by having sexual relations.
2. The statistics of cancer and Herpes must be clarified.

3. The importance of regular Pap tests.
4. Cervical cancer in surface tissues and in deeper tissues and other concerns.

1. YOU CANNOT TRANSMIT CANCER BY HAVING SEXUAL RELATIONS

David, you said that you gave cancer to your fiancée because you had sex when you had active Herpes lesions.

The Herpes virus can certainly be transferred to your fiancée, as I've pointed out many times already. You can give her Herpes. But that does not mean she has, or even is going to get, cancer of the cervix.

At the present time, we do not know what is the cause of cancer of the cervix. It is possible that the Herpes virus may be the cause but most authorities believe it is some other factor. Some authorities feel that there is a rare possibility that the Herpes virus might be altered during replication in such a way that malignant changes might occur in cells that were particularly susceptible. These cells might then have the ability to proliferate in an abnormal manner.

The theory of the cause of increased cancer of the cervix that makes the most sense to me is the one which argues that the Herpes virus first helps to destroy the defensive mechanism of the cells of the cervix in susceptible individuals. Then the cause of cancer of the cervix, whether it is Herpes virus, another virus, or whatever, can attack and overpower those cells.

David, there are several different kinds of cancer that also seem to be increased in frequency when they are related to the Herpes virus. Cancer of the prostate gland and cancer of the penis are more frequent cancers in men. Cancers of the tissues of the lip, mouth, and pharynx are associated with Herpes Type 1 in both

196

women and men. An interesting aside, David, is that every one of these cancers, except cancer of the penis, also are reported to occur more frequently in persons who smoke.

It must be noted that these are statistical associations only. We do not know the cause of cancer of these organs.

2. THE STATISTICS OF CANCER AND HERPES MUST BE CLARIFIED

We must be clear about what we are saying in the relationship of cancer and Herpes virus disease.

One thing we are saying is that HERPES EVIDENCE IS FOUND FREQUENTLY IN THE CERVICAL TISSUES OF WOMEN WHO HAVE CANCER OF THE CERVIX.

Another thing we are saying is that CANCER OF THE CERVIX IS FOUND MORE FREQUENTLY IN WOMEN WHO HAVE A HISTORY OF HAVING HERPES.

What we are NOT saying is that all women who get Herpes will have cancer of the cervix.

The statistics tell us that the rate of cancer of the cervix is eight times higher among women who have a history of Herpes than it is among women who do not have such a history. That is scary but it does not mean that all women who have Herpes will develop cancer of the cervix. I have stated the same thing twice so that it will not be misunderstood. What these statistics do tell us loud and clear is that we must be extremely careful to find every case of cancer of the cervix before it is neglected.

Another fact that the statisticians tell us is that certain women have a greater chance to develop cancer of the cervix. Other women do not seem to develop cancer as frequently. These facts do not consider Herpes in their compilation. However, when we think of cancer of the cervix these classes must be considered.

Women having a higher incidence of cancer of the cervix are:

Women age 35 to 60
Women who began sexual intercourse at an early age
Women of the lower socioeconomic status
Women with poor genital hygiene

Women who have a lower incidence of cancer of the cervix are:

Women below the age of 30 years
Celibate women such as nuns
Jewish women (indicated by some researchers)
Women who have never borne children

David, please hear what I am indicating. It is simply that a higher percent of the women in the high incidence group will develop cancer. I am NOT saying that all women in that group will have it.

When we calculate the frequency of women who are in the high incidence group with those that have a history of Herpes infection then there is cause to be very careful about preventing or finding further problems.

3. THE IMPORTANCE OF REGULAR PAP TESTS

The above information is frightening. One case of cancer is too many. Many cases are a disaster. But there is hope in the Papanicolaou's stain test! This test is easy and inexpensive. It is reliable and tells us early of the presence of cancer cells in the tissue.

ANY WOMAN WHO HAS HAD HERPES OR WHOSE SEXUAL PARTNER HAS HAD HERPES SHOULD HAVE A PAP TEST TWICE A YEAR.

Cancer of the cervix is curable if it is found early. I'll say it again. CANCER OF THE CERVIX IS CURABLE IF IT IS FOUND EARLY.

A patient who has had Herpes does not need to panic. She does not need to give up, to say nothing can be done. On the contrary, she must not give up but she must have examinations twice a year and make sure that a Pap test is done. The patient and her doctor must be aware that she is in a higher risk group and be alert to institute comprehensive study and treatment for cancer of the cervix if the Pap test is positive.

If there is anything in this book that you want to remember, please let this be part of it. Any woman who has had genital Herpes, or whose sexual partner has had Herpes, should have a Pap test every six months.

There are no exceptions to this rule unless you have had a hysterectomy and have no cervix. Even if your gynecologist feels it is not necessary, please make arrangements to get such a test. Most of the time the gynecologist's opinion is true, but in this matter of Herpes, be on the conservative side.

The reason I am so strong about this advice lies in the next sub-topic.

4. CERVICAL CANCER IN SURFACE TISSUES AND CERVICAL CANCER IN DEEPER TISSUES AND OTHER CANCERS

The cervix is a doughnut-shaped structure which is the lower end of the uterus. The main strength of the circular muscle fibers which make up the cervix act as the large valve that closes the lower end of the womb. The muscle is covered by a layer of cardboard-carton-like cells similar to those which were described lining the inside of the mouth.

This anatomical concept is important, for the cervix might be likened to a roll of paper towels which are purchased at the supermarket. Those towels are covered by plastic and completely protected.

Let us imagine that a drop of pickled beet juice, that bright maroon liquid, falls on the roll of toweling every second. This goes on for hours or days and nothing happens to the paper towel. It is still good: dry and white. After a week of the dripping, one drop sneaks through a tiny hole in the plastic—and suddenly much of the toweling is stained red.

The illustration holds with tissues of the cervix. Cancer can attack the surface box-like cells. These cuboid guard-layer cells resist invasion with great persistence for months or even years. The cancer is only present on the exterior surface of the cervix and at that time is called carcinoma in situ (cancer that is confined to the site of origin without invasion of neighboring tissues). However, after a long time, the cancer can break through the guard layer and get into the deeper tissues where, like the beet juice, its spread is much more difficult to control.

We are not, at this time, able to estimate when the breakthrough will occur. Waiting too long may be disastrous.

Pap tests alert patient and doctor that something is happening to the tissue and cancer cells are present. If the basement layer has not been penetrated, complete cure can be effected by treatment of the cervix. It is possible that a hysterectomy may be performed to assure removal of the entire problem tissue.

After the cancer has broken through the surface layer it is much more difficult to control and the cure ratio decreases. If the cancer has spread to the next level of defense, the lymph nodes, the situation becomes even more critical.

Other cancers, though much more rare, are similarly related to Herpes. The earlier they are found, the better the chance of recovery.

Cancer of the prostate could be increased in patients who have a history of Herpes. A special class like that which I cited for the incidence of women having cancer of the cervix is also apparent in this problem. Black men have a much higher rate of prostatic cancer than do others. All men who have a history of Herpes should be checked at least yearly. Black men with a Herpes history should be checked at least twice yearly because of the higher risk ratio.

Cancer of the mouth resembles cancer of the cervix in many ways. Both areas are lined by similar tissues. As I stated under the section on cervical cancer, the first sign is a premalignant lesion, one that may develop into cancer in the future. A premalignant lesion also is common in the mouth. Herpes virus Type 1 is often found when there is cancer of the mouth. The research has not been great into this phenomenon yet, but the possibility is strong that a relationship may occur in cancer of the mouth as in cancer of the cervix.

Though the treatment of cancer is productive if found early, preventing Herpes in the first place is far more effective. This process, as I have related, takes hard work on the part of the patient, but is worth the trouble many times over.

Chapter 17

SO WHAT?

Dr. Joe Robertson, this final chapter is written especially for you. It's written to summarize for the millions of patients who are afflicted with Herpes what I have been trying to say throughout the book. What is this disease we call Herpes? What causes it? How can it be prevented? How can I tell if I've got it? How can it be treated?

All these things, Dr. Robertson, I want to condense into a few pages.

This disease is epidemic. That's not hard to realize from where each of us have our interest and activity—in medicine. It is all around us. My wife, Jean, has been helping me by reading and editing, and took the chapter on Triggers to the beauty parlor to read while she was having her hair done. Inadvertently she left the papers there when she left. When she returned a few days later to ask for it, the manager said, "Is that yours?"

"Yes," Jean replied, "my husband is writing a book on Herpes. I hope it didn't embarrass you."

"Well, it was quite frank. I asked three of my customers if it was theirs. They all said no, but they all read it avidly and asked where they could buy the book. Because they all had Herpes." And this was in swank Newport Beach, California.

Perhaps the most surprising thing about it, Joe, is the

way it has crept upon us. It began almost like the tid
until suddenly, it's a tsunami. As you remember, one c
the classic textbooks which we used in medical schoo'
was Novak's *Gynecology*. I reviewed several edition
and in 1956 the word "Herpes" was not mentioned
There were two paragraphs in the following editio
about ten years later. The last revision carries a whol
section.

How did it happen so quickly? There must be some
thing coincidental to cause the spread of a disease tha
was well described 200 years ago. This raises question
that we cannot answer as yet. Is the pill partly responsi
ble? Smoking? Increased sexual activity? Different sex
ual styles? We shall begin to unravel the snarl soon be
cause the amount of research is enormous, an
increasing. And yet to further complicate the tangle
some of the results of excellent researchers produce dia
metrically different answers.

There are some things of which we are sure. The dis
ease is caused by a virus that has two separate strains
Each causes a set of slightly different symptoms. Th
strains can be interchangeable as far as the anatom
goes.

Generally, the Type 1 virus causes lesions of the lips
keratitis, canker sores, and ulcers in the mouth an
pharynx, skin lesions, and encephalitis.

Herpes Type 2 usually causes genital lesions in botl
women and men. These painful sores are often multipl
and usually extremely tender to the touch. It is th
usual cause of infection in the newborn.

The sores produced by either Type 1 or Type 2 las
about a week to ten days and gradually disappear. Th
lesions remind me of a first or second degreee burn
and they progress in a similar manner.

One of the most important things to remember is tha
the lesions often occur inside the vagina and frequentl
do not cause pain. A diligent search, a Pap test, and

culture must be completed on all women who have vulvar lesions or a history of having had sexual relations with a partner who had Herpes.

Joe, one of the most important contributions to the health of the people we serve is to make sure that each woman has a Pap test every year, or, if she has had Herpes or been exposed to Herpes, twice yearly. She should have the frequent Pap tests until she reaches age 60 at least. After that one per year will probably be sufficient.

The virus that causes Herpes is a difficult one to deal with. It gets into the body in one of a myriad of ways, through a break in the skin, through the intestinal tract, and even upstream through the urinary tract. This ultramicroscopic structure is a DNA virus and as such may control the life force of any cell it infects. It can cause the destruction of many of the defensive cells of the Immune System; T-lymphocytes, B-lymphocytes, and macrophages to name but a few. When this happens the defenses are weakened. The body is less able to cope with the attack upon it and may be unable to keep the virus under control.

If the body is in a weakened and vulnerable state, any additional strain may be enough of a trigger to break down the usual defenses and open up an outbreak of Herpes lesions.

Tell your patients that there are myriads of triggers. Probably every person can think of some that are the things that cause an effect upon them. I know that walnuts and macadamia nuts are triggers for canker sores for me. It is important for your patients to think seriously about that so that those things that are triggers can be avoided.

The most frequently named trigger is stress. No doubt, a big factor in many Herpes recurrences. Others beside food are sunshine, fatigue, sex, athletics, menstrual periods, the seasons, trauma, and serious debilitating disease.

The patient usually wants to know how they got the disease. This is a problem, for the answer may threaten the breakup of a marital relationship. I am convinced that some Herpes can be contracted innocently. Unless I'm very naive, and an ex-army Veneral Disease Control officer isn't known for naiveté, I have cared for patients who had such an event. I estimate perhaps 10% may have an initial episode from a trigger of severe stress or innocent contact such as a toilet seat. How else would patients with debilitating disease develop Herpes? For we can be fairly sure they have had no sexual contact.

One of the things that I believe should be explained to your patients is the Immune Response. The concept is very important to help patients understand how every single self-help that they may use to assist their own resistance, may ward off or prevent an attack. Keeping the virus particles dormant in the nerve tissue is our most important treatment at this time.

I do not know which of the several short diagnostic tests for Herpes that you may use, Joe, but most of them are usually satisfactory. However, I still rely on the older measures, cultures of the virus from the moisture of the lesions, and Pap smears to identify the multinucleated giant cells. Many fine clinical laboratories like the ones in your area can complete these tests in a short time with high reliability.

Probably the most dependable aspect of diagnosis is your own acute clinical sense. Herpes presents many pictures but usually they are typical. Don't forget that you are a trained doctor, Joe. Your wide experience is the basis for the calm and clear counsel that you can give to a frightened and nervous patient when you must make the diagnosis of Herpes. Study all you can about the disease, attend the refresher courses, and relate what you know of the disease to your patients and to your staff. The nurses and receptionists working with you often are the ones to whom the patients relate, so bring them up to date on the many aspects of the disease. The treatment is twofold. We must use every weapon in our armamentarium to help the patient combat the ravages of the virus. In the present state of the art probably the most work in fighting the disease lies on the shoulders of the patients.

They should be carefully counselled about the old-time sterile techniques. Remember those things we were taught in medical school—before the discovery of penicillin by Dr. Fleming. We had to wash and wash and wash. Clothing was protected, linen was held separate until it could be carefully laundered. In some instances we gowned before visiting a patient. Drinking glasses and dishes were handled separately.

We have to return to those days of hard work. If the patients don't work to keep the epidemic under control, it will not be deterred and will rage on unchecked. Prevention and the care it entails is the most important weapon that is now authorized.

Joe, many treatments have been found to be ineffective. When that happens, it is most frustrating to be a doctor and have to tell patients you don't have anything to help them.

I do not advise multiple smallpox vaccinations, as the chance of generalized vaccinia far outweighs the apparent benefit derived from such a series.

Ultraviolet treatments make no sense to me at all, for sunshine is one of the most vigorous triggers. Why subject the patient to more of the thing that may have been the cause of the problem in the first place?

In my experience the several dyes and photoinactivation have little benefit.

The one hope that I can hold out is that there are new treatments down the road a little way, Joe. The

FDA will subject them to a long period of testing before their approval is granted.

The arabinosides and IDU do not seem to be of great help for local treatment except in the problem of keratitis.

Acyclovir has promise but testing has yet to be completed.

Interferon is available in such small quantities and is so expensive that it has rarely been used for uncomplicated Herpes studies.

It would seem that vaccinations would be an answer, but the complexity of the virus itself has made vaccines difficult to perfect.

The drug we were testing is available in much of the world. It has no apparent side effects and has caused no birth defects. It seems to be an effective medication. It is not yet authorized by the Food and Drug Administration. We must wait.

Herpes in pregnancy remains a serious problem and a growing one. It is incumbent on us all to try to prevent mothers who have active lesions from delivering in the normal manner, through the vagina. Caesarean Section is the main method of circumventing the vaginal route. This must be explained to patients and doctors so that great care can be taken to test the vaginal tissues for virus shedding and active lesions.

Isolation techniques need to be provided for the babies whose mothers or fathers have ever had Herpes. The devastating effect of the virus upon a newborn infant is to be avoided at all costs.

Friends, relatives, nurses, and doctors must be educated to stay away from the baby if they have Herpes lesions of any kind. Fever blisters are included in that statement.

There is some sort of relationship between Herpes and cancer that has yet to be understood fully. Cancer of the cervix occurs more frequently in women who have had Herpes. A debate is in progress among authorities as to whether the Herpes virus or something else is the cause of the problem.

Our job, Dr. Robertson, is to make sure that we find any such cancer at the earliest moment. Cancer of the cervix is curable if found early, before the basal layer of the cervical tissue is penetrated. Pap tests every six months will alert physicians, health professionals, and nurse practitioners, that a problem of malignancy exists and treatment should be instituted.

Don't forget that Pap tests can be used in any area of the body to locate Herpes and possibly to avert malignancy. We do find increased chance of cancer of the prostate, the penis, and the oral cavity in persons who have a history of Herpes, so it is incumbent upon us to be vigilant to find lesions in any area of the body.

Joe, the following chart is one which I have prepared. It summarizes my feeling about who seems to be more susceptible to developing Herpes. The material is based on the research study and on my observations. I am a little hesitant to open this to the public, for I do not want to be in the same position as the writer in the popular magazine that seemed to give the impression that every woman who has Herpes will have cancer of the cervix. As you know, this is not the case, but some people did not understand what has been said. In this list I am trying to separate classes of persons more apt to develop the disease from classes less likely to develop it.

Classes of persons developing
Herpes simplex virus disease

More likely to develop Herpes	Less likely to develop Herpes

Type 1

Fair-skinned persons	Dark-skinned persons
Exposure to sun	Protection from sun
Smokers	Non-smokers
Ages 4–15	Over age 30
Fever	Healthy
Debilitating disease	Health
Diet high in argenine	Diet low in argenine
Diet low in lysine	Diet high in lysine

Type 2

Nations with promiscuous mores	Less promiscuous mores
Many sexual partners	Celibates, nuns, etc.
Stressful life	Well-adjusted life
Smokers	Non-smokers
Age 18 to 30	Under 18, over 30
Borderline physical or chronic illness	Good physical health
Menstrual women	Menopausal women
Women on birth control pills	No birth control pills
High argenine diet	Low argenine diet
Low lysine diet	High lysine diet

This list is in generalities only. A person should attempt to work from the left-hand list toward the right-hand list wherever it is possible.

So what, Joe? You asked me what do I tell patients about Herpes. What advice do I give? I guess this is it.

Herpes is a nasty disease—caused by a complicated and frustrating virus. It acts differently in various individuals. But it can be beaten.

To accomplish defeat of the virus takes work. Work on the part of the patient. It involves relearning tech-

210

niques of keeping oneself clean and pure. Of keeping clothing, dishes, and other personal items separated from others in the home or environment. It involves being ever vigilant to avoid triggers that will set off an episode of the infection, for it is during the time of active lesions that the disease spreads most easily.

One excellent source of assistance for Herpes, Joe, to which you can refer your patients is called HELP. It is a program of the American Social Health Association. There are chapters in over 30 cities to provide current developments involving Herpes, and to answer questions via a national hotline. The address is:

HELP/ASHA
P.O. Box 100
Palo Alto, California 94302.

There is hope, too, for the development of new medications for the disease. In other parts of the world the research is progressing. And here, too. It is a matter of time before we will have the answer to Herpes virus disease.

GLOSSARY

ANAEROBIC   Organisms that live and thrive in the absence of oxygen.

AMINO ACID   A complicated organic molecule, usually a component of food.

AMNIOTIC FLUID   The water which surrounds the infant inside the uterus.

ANTIGEN   Blood components that react to an antibody or a lymphocyte.

ANTIBODIES   A complex molecule that has a specific amino acid which reacts only with another specific antigen.

ANUS   The valve at the terminal end of the intestine.

ARGENINE   An amino acid, seems to promote Herpes.

ASYMPTOMATIC CARRIERS   Those persons who harbor the virus or other causes of disease within their body. They are capable of transmitting the disease but they do not have any symptoms.

AUTOINOCULATION   The spread of an infection to one's own body from another part of one's own body.

AVASCULAR   A rare area of the anatomy where few capillaries exist and where rare blood cells are found. Nerve tissue is of this type.

BLEB   A large vesicle or blister filled with fluid.

BLOODSTREAM   The immense series of blood vessels, arteries, capillaries, and veins that circulate blood.

BORIC ACID   A weak antiseptic salt, usually used as a solution.

BULLA   A large vesicle or blister.

BURROW'S SOLUTION   A topical solution for the skin.

CANKER SORES Fever blisters, cold sores.

CARCINOMA IN SITU Cancer, usually of the cervix, which has not broken through the basement (guard) layer of the tissue.

CAUDA EQUINA The nerve tissue in which the Herpes virus Type 2 probably lies dormant.

CELL A microscopic mass of protoplasm wrapped in a semipermeable membrane, containing a nucleus. It is capable of reacting with other cells in the fundamental functions of life.

CELLULAR IMMUNE FUNCTIONS The processes in the immune protection by the cells of the blood and lymph stream.

CAESAREAN SECTION A major surgical operation to deliver a baby.

CERVIX The lower part of the uterus. It protects the womb and is located in the upper part of the vagina.

CHANCRE The sore of syphilis, first stage.

CHROMOSOME The part of the cell nucleus that divides equally and determines the genetic destiny of the cell.

CLITORIS A sensitive stimulatory organ located anterior to the vagina.

COLD SORE Fever blister, Herpes labialis.

COMMITTED CELLS Cells which work to destroy specific cells for which they are programmed.

CORTISONE A hormone of the adrenal cortex.

CRATER The walls which surround the ulcer of Herpes.

C.S.U.F. California State University, Fullerton.

CULTURE (laboratory) Artificial growth in the laboratory of tissues, bacteria, or viruses, etc.

CYSTITIS Urinary tract infection of women and men.

DEBILITATING DISEASE Diseases which sap the patient's strength, such as cancer.

DERMATOME A delineated nerve distribution on the surface of the skin.

DERMIS The growing, sensitive, inner layer of the skin.

DODERLEIN'S BACILLI The normal defensive bacteria of the vagina.

DORMANT VIRUS PARTICLES Virions that are latent in nerve tissue.

DNA A complicated nucleic acid that is the life force of a cell.

DOUBLE-BLIND STUDY A research study in which researchers do not know until the study is ended which patient or subject is receiving an active treament or which a placebo.

EFFECTOR CELLS Cells which combat toxic antigens that poison the system.

ELECTRON-MICROSCOPE A device for viewing matter smaller than ordinary microscopes can detect.

ENCEPHALITIS Inflammation of the brain.

EPIDERMIS The outermost, avascular layer of the skin.

EPISODIC Occurring at usual or irregular intervals.

ERYTHROCYTES Red blood cells.

EXUDATE The serum from sores of all kinds, Herpes and others.

FEVER BLISTER A cold sore, Herpes labialis.

FIBER Roughage, a most important part of the diet.

FORCHET The area between the vagina and the anus.

GENETICS The study of heredity.

GONORRHEA The very common venereal disease.

GYNECOLOGIST A physician who deals with the diseases of women.

HERPES The disease discussed in this book.

HERPES ZOSTER Shingles, a nerve irritation caused by varicella virus.

HERPETIC Relating to Herpes.

HYDROCORTISONE A refined derivative of cortisone.

HYMEN The fragile tissue covering of the lower end of the vaginal opening.

HYMENAL RING The remnant of the hymen.

IMMUNE RESPONSE The teamwork of the body to fight a disease.

IMMUNOPOTENTIATORS A class of drugs that boost the Immune Response.

INFECTIOUS Capable of transmitting disease.

INFLAMMATION A red area of the skin caused by infection or trauma.

KERATITIS Inflammation of the cornea of the eye. May be caused by the Herpes virus.

LABIA The lips of the vagina.

LACTOBACILLAE The normal defensive bacteria of the vagina.

LATENT PERIOD The period of many diseases when nothing happens but the causative agent is ready to become active.

LESION A sore or small ulcer.

LYMPH GLAND OR NODE An anatomical accumulation of lymphoid tissue. A defensive area of the body.

LYMPHOCYTES White blood cells which neutralize antigenic substances which enter the body.

LYMPH STREAM A companion system of vessels to the bloodstream. Lymph circulates throughout the body and is one of the vital defense mechanisms.

LYSINE An amino acid which helps prevent Herpes.

MACROPHAGES White blood cells that are the street-sweepers of the bloodstream.

MATURATION The process of development.

MEMBRANES The covering of the bag of waters which breaks during the birth process.

MEMORY CELLS Messenger cells which call up the reserves in the fight of the Immune Response.

MONS VENERIS The rounded area of the pubis, where the hair is.

NUCLEUS/NUCLEI The central portion of tissue cells and other cells. The portion of the cell which contains chromosomes.

OBSTETRICIAN A physician who assists in the delivery of babies.

OPHTHALMOLOGIST A physician who treats diseases of the eye.

ORAL-GENITAL SEX The act of oral titillation of the genital area.

PAP TEST The Papanicolaou's stain test for cancer. Also used effectively in the diagnosis of Herpes.

PEDIATRICIAN A physician who treats diseases of children.

PENIS The male sex organ.

PERINEUM The pelvic floor in men and women.

PHA The test for Immune Response level.

PHAGOCYTIC CELLS The streetsweepers of the blood-stream.

PHOTOINACTIVATION A treatment of Herpes using light and dyes.

PHYTOHEMAGGLUTININ Test for the Immune Response level. The PHA.

PLACEBO EFFECT The result of improvement when the patient thinks he or she is receiving a beneficial treatment when they are not.

PLACEBO A fake medicine, one without chemical effect.

PRIMARY CASES Original cases of a disease.

PSYCHIATRIST A physician who treats diseases of the mind.

PSYCHOLOGIST A person trained in the science that deals with the mind and behavior.

REPLICATE The process by which a virus reproduces its own kind or a variant.

REPORTABLE DISEASE Disease which health professionals report to public health resources in order to facilitate control.

RNA A nucleic acid that is the messenger between DNA and the protein-forming system.

SCROTUM The sack which contains the testicles.

SECONDARY CASES Recurrences of a disease. Repeated episodes.

SERUM The clear fluid that seeps from a lesion.

SHINGLES Herpes zoster.

STEM CELLS The basic undifferentiated cells of the bloodstream. At first it is undetermined what cells they will eventually become.

STEROID A hormone, cortisone or hydrocortisone.

STRESS Mental tension.

SYPHILIS A venereal disease caused by a spirochete.

TARGET CELLS Are marked for destruction because they have been contaminated.

T-LYMPHOCYTES Thymic defensive cells.

TROCHE A lozenge.

TRAUMA An injury to tissues or psyche.

TRIGEMINAL NERVE A nerve in the region of the jaw in which the Herpes virus Type 1 lies dormant.

TRIGGER An event, substance, disease, or stress that sets off Herpes episode.

TUMESCENCE Swelling.

ULCER The typical painful crater of Herpes. The skin lesion of the disease.

ULTRAMICROSCOPIC Smaller than capable of being detected by an ordinary microscope.

ULTRAVIOLET RAYS The sun's rays which may be harmful to some.

URETHRA The tube through which urine flows out of the body. It is located anterior to the vagina in women and in the penis in men. Semen is also discharged from the urethra of men during the sex act.

VACCINATIONS The process of inoculation of a similar bacteria or virus into the body in order to immunize against a more virulent disease agent.

VACCINIA A generalized eruption of vaccinations after smallpox vaccinations.

VAGINA The tube that leads from the cervix to the external female genital area. It is the female part involved in the sex act.

VARICELLA Chicken pox.

VESICLE A serum-filled small bleb.

VIRICIDES Drugs that kill or prevent a virus from replicating.

VIRION An individual virus particle.

VIRUS An ultramicroscopic agent of disease.

VIRUS SHEDDING The detectable virus in moisture of various parts of the body. Evidence of infection.

VULVA The external genital area of women and girls.

WATER The amniotic sac or the "bag of waters."

WHITLOW A Herpes infection of the finger.

BIBLIOGRAPHY

American Academy of Pediatrics, Committee on Fetus and Newborn, Committee on Infectious Diseases. 1980. Perinatal herpes simplex virus infections, Pediatrics, vol. 66, no. 1: 147–49.

Amstey, M.S. Herpes virus (letter). *Obstetrics and Gynecology*, vol. 52. no. 5: 640, 1978.

Azulay, R.D., and Azulay, E. 1975. Emprego de un novo antivirotico, isoprinosine, no herpes simples e no herpes zoster. *Revista Braseleira De Medicina*, vol. 32, no. 2: 105–09.

Biro, C.E. 1972. Clinical investigation with isoprinosine in patients with herpes simplex and herpes zoster. *El Medico* (Mexico), vol. 5: 75–82.

Boles-Carenini, B., Grignolo, F.M., Brogliatte, B., and Lo Presti, L. 1978. *Therapeutic/Treatment With Isoprinosine (Delalande) of Ocular Diseases Caused by Herpes Simplex.* Turino: Oculistics Clinic of the University of Turino, Italy.

Bradshaw, L.J., Sumner, H.L., Wickett, W.H., Jr., and Correia, E.B. 1980. Immunological and clinical studies on herpes simplex patients treated with inosiplex. 4th

218

International Congress of Immunology, Paris France, 21–26, July 1980. (Abstracts.)

Bradshaw, L.J., and Sumner, H.L. 1977. In vitro studies on cell-mediated immunity in patients treated with inosiplex for herpes virus infection. Annals of the New York Academy of Sciences, Vol. 284: 190–96.

Brann, A.W., Chairman, Committee on Fetus and Newborn, et al., and Mortimer, E.A., Jr., Chairman, Committee on Infectious Diseases, 1980. Perinatal herpes simplex virus infections, *Pediatrics*, vol. 66, no. 1: 147–49.

Breen, J.L., and Smith, C.I. 1981. Sexually transmitted diseases, Part 1. *The Female Patient*, vol. 6, no. 7: 12–18.

Genital herpes. 1980. *British Medical Journal*, vol. 280, no. 6228: 1335–36.

Buge, A., et al. 1979. Les aspects tomodensitometriques (c.t. scan) des encephalites aigues necrosantes herpetiques. *Review of Neurology* (Paris), vol. 135, no. 5: 401–406.

Chang, T., Fiumara, N., and Weinstein, L. 1973. Treatment of herpes progenitalis with isoprinosine. Paper presented at the Thirteenth Interscience Conference on Antimicrobial Agents, 21, Sept. 1973, at Tufts-New England Medical Center.

Chang, T. 1977. Genital herpes and type 1 herpesvirus hominis. *Journal of the American Medical Association*, vol. 238, no. 2: 155.

Corey, L., et al. 1978. Ineffectiveness of topical ether for

for the treatment of genital herpes simplex virus infection. *The New England Journal of Medicine*, vol. 299, no. 5: 237–39.

Corey, L., Reeves, W.C., and Holmes, K.K. 1978. Cellular immune response in genital herpes simplex virus infection. *The New England Journal of Medicine*, vol. 299, no. 18: 986–91.

Corey, L., et al. 1979. Effect of isoprinosine on the cellular immune response in initial genital herpes virus infection. *Clinical Research* (Abstract.)

Costa, J.C., and Rabson, A.S. 1979. Latent infection by herpes simplex virus. *Pathology Annual*, vol. 14, part 2: 61–68.

Cousins, N. 1979. *Anatomy of an Illness as Perceived by the Patient*. New York: W.W. Norton and Company.

Crow, T.J. 1978. Viral causes of psychiatric disease. *Postgraduate Medical Journal*, vol. 54: 763–67.

Feldman, S., Hayies, F., Chaudhary, S., and Ossi, M. 1978. Inosiplex for localized herpes zoster in childhood cancer patients: preliminary controlled study. *Antimicrobial Agents and Chemotherapy*, vol. 14, no. 3: 495–97.

Ferruti, M., and Acquisto, R. 1978. L'isoprinosina, nuovo virustatico, nel trattamento dell'herpes genitalis. Revista di patologia e Clinica, vol. 33, no. 2: 82–104, Ospedale Bassini, Milan, Italy.

Glogau, R.G. 1980. How I treat herpes, *Medical Times*, vol. 108, no. 3: 66–68.

Gordon, P., Ronsen, B., and Brown, E. 1974. Anti-herpesvirus action of isoprinosine. *Antimicrobial Agents and Chemotherapy*, vol. 5, no. 2: 153–60.

Griffith, R.S., Norris, A.L., and Kagan, C. 1978. A multi-centered study of lysine therapy in herpes simplex infection. *Dermatologica*, vol. 156: 257–67.

Guinan, M.E., et al. 1980. Topical ether and herpes simplex labialis. *Journal of the American Medical Association*, vol. 243, no. 10: 1059–61.

Hadden, J.W. 1977. The action of immunopotentiators in vitro on lymphocyte and macrophage activation. Memorial Sloan Kettering Cancer Center, New York, N.Y.

Hensleigh, P.A., Glover, D.B., and Cannon, M. 1979. Systemic Herpesvirus hominis in pregnancy. *The Journal of Reproductive Medicine*, vol. 22, no. 3: 171–76.

Hittleman, R. 1969. Yoga: 28 day exercise plan. New York: Workman Publishing Co.

Huttenlocher, P.R., and Mattson, R.H. 1979. Isoprinosine in subacute sclerosing panencephalitis. *Neurology*, vol. 29: 763–71.

Jeansson, S., and Molin, L. 1974. On the occurrence of genital herpes simplex virus infection. *Acta Dermatovener* (Stockholm), vol. 54: 479–85.

Kagan, C. 1974. Lysine therapy for herpes simplex, *The Lancet*. (Communication.)

Kaplan, A.S. 1973. The herpesviruses. New York and London: Academic Press.

Kernbaum, S., and Hauchecorne, J. 1981. Administration

of levodopa for relief of herpes zoster pain. *Journal of the American Medical Association*, vol. 246, no. 2: 132–34.

Kibrick, S. 1979. Herpes simplex virus in breast milk. *Pediatrics*, vol. 64, no. 3. (Letter.)

Kibrick, S. 1980. Herpes simplex infection at term. What to do with mother, newborn, and nursery personnel. *Journal of the American Medical Association*, vol. 243, no. 2: 157–60.

King, R.L. 1979. Herpes simplex encephalitis in pregnancy. *American Journal of Obstetrics and Gynecology*, vol. 135, no. 8: 1114–15.

Kruger, G.G., et al. Treatment of recurrent herpes simplex labialis (HSL) with levamisole. Presented at 18th Interscience Conference on Antimicrobial Agents and Chemotherapy, Oct. 1-4, 1978. Atlanta, Ga. (Abstract.)

Little, J.W. 1979. Oral cancer and herpes simplex virus— a review, St. Louis, Mo.: C.V. Mosby Co.

Light, I.J. 1979. Postnatal acquisition of herpes simplex virus by the newborn infant: A review of the literature. *Pediatrics*, vol. 63, no. 3: 480–82.

Luby, J.P. 1979. Antivirals with clinical potential. The Year Book Medical Publishers, Inc., Chicago. p. 229.

Macnab, J.C. 1980. Carcinoma of the penis and cervix. *Lancet*, vol. 2., no. 8198: 805. (Letter.)

Marks, M.I. 1974. Variables influencing the vitro susceptibilities of herpes simplex viruses to antiviral drugs.

Antimicrobial Agents and Chemotherapy, vol. 6, no. 1: 34–48.

Marks, M.I. 1975. Evaluation of four antiviral agents in the treatment of herpes simplex encephalitis in a rat model. *The Journal of Infectious Diseases*, vol. 131, no. 1: 11–16.

Merrigan, T.C. 1976. Efficacy of adenine arabinoside in herpes zoster. Editorial, *The New England Journal of Medicine*, vol. 294, no. 22: 1233–34.

Muracciole, J.C., Vilarino, J.S., and Vilarino, M.A. 1973. Tratamiento de las lesiones virales—herpes simple—herpes zoster herpangina—con el agente antiviral isoprinosine. *Revista del circulo Arg. de Odontologia*, vol. 35, no. 3: 22–35.

Nahmias, A.J., and Norrild, B. 1979. Herpes simplex viruses, 1 and 2—Basic and clinical aspects. *Dermatology*, vol. 25, no. 10: 1–49.

Nahmias, A.J. 1981. Herpes from womb to tomb. Lecture, presented at International Virology Symposium, 9, Oct. 1981, Anaheim, Calif.

Nahmias, A.J. 1980. Herpes simplex virus infection: problems and prospects as perceived by a peripatetic pediatrician. *The Yale Journal of Biology and Medicine*, vol. 53, no. 1: 47–54.

Nahmias, A.J., and Roizman, B. 1973. Infection with herpes simplex viruses 1 and 2. *The New England Journal of Medicine*, vol. 289, no. 15: 781–89.

Novak and Novak. 1956, 1966, and 1975 editions. Textbook of gynecology. Williams and Wilkins. Baltimore.

Oill, P.A., and Mishell, D.R., Jr. 1980. Symposium on adolescent gynecology and endocrinology, Part III: Venereal diseases in adolescents and contraception in teenagers. *The Western Journal of Medicine,* vol. 132: 39–48.

Orren, A., et al. 1981. Increased susceptibility to herpes simplex virus infections in children with acute measles. *Infection and Immunity,* vol. 31, no. 1: 1–6.

Peck, M.S. 1978. The road less traveled. New York: Simon and Schuster.

Poirier, R.H. 1980. Nerpetic ocular infections in childhood. *Archives of Ophthalmology,* vol. 98: 704–6.

Rapp, F. 1980. Virology and cancer. *Preventive Medicine,* vol. 9: 244–51.

Rapp, R., and Jerkofsky, M. 1973. The herpesviruses: Persistent and latent infections. Chapter 9: 171–289. New York: Academic Press Inc.

Rawls, W.E. 1973. Herpes simplex virus. Chapter 10: 291–325. New York: Academic Press Inc.

Sabin, A.B. 1981. Immunization, evaluation of some currently available and prospective vaccines. *Journal of the American Medical Association,* vol. 246, no. 3: 236–41.

Sabin, A.B., and Tarro, G. 1973. Herpes simplex and herpes genitalis viruses in etiology of some human cancers. Proceedings, National Academy of Science, vol. 70, no. 11: 3225–29.

Schreiner, R.L., Kleiman, M.B., and Gresham, E.L. 1979. Maternal oral herpes: Isolation policy, *Pediatrics*, vol. 63, no. 2: 247–49.

Sequiera, L.W., et al. 1979. Detection of herpes simplex viral genome in brain tissue. *The Lancet*, vol. 2. no. 8143: 609–12.

Sexually Transmitted Diseases Bulletin, 1981. Vol. 1, nos. 1—4.

Shillitoe, E.J., Silverman, S., Jr. 1979. Oral cancer and herpes simplex virus—a review. *Oral Surgery*, vol. 48, no. 3: 216–24.

Shklar, G. 1981. Common oral mucosal diseases, *Medical Times*, vol. 109, no. 6.

Sinha, S.K. 1979. An overview of significant research on viral infections of the foetus associated with congenital defects and mental deficiencies. *Journal of Mental Deficiency Research*, vol. 23, no. 3: 207–12.

Sparling, P.F. 1979. Current problems in sexually transmitted diseases. *Advances in Internal Medicine*, vol. 24: 203–28.

Spruance, S.L., et al. 1978. Treatment of herpes simplex labialis with adenine arabinoside-5'-monophosphate (ARA-AMP). Presented at 18th Interscience Conference on Antimicrobial Agents and Chemotherapy, 1–4, Oct. 1978, Atlanta, Ga. (Abstract.)

Sternberg, T.H., and Ruiz, E.M. 1972. The treatment of herpes zoster and herpes simplex with isoprinosine, *La Prenza Medica Mexicana*, vol. 37, nos. 3 and 4: 159–60.

Tejani, N., et al. 1979. Subclinical herpes simplex genitalis infections in the perinatal period. *American Journal of Obstetrics and Gynecology*, vol. 135, no. 4: 547.

Tenaglia, R., and Carcano del Campo, C. Tentiva de prevencion de la queratoconjuntivitis epidemica en medicina laboral. *Medicina y Terapeutica* vol. 1 no. 9: 403–08, December 1973. (Argentina.)

Thong, Y.H., et al. 1975. Depressed specific cell-mediated immunity to herpes simplex virus type 1 in patients with recurrent herpes labialis. *Infection and Immunity*, vol. 12, no. 1: 76–80.

Whitley, R.J., Nahmias, A.J., et al. 1980. The natural history of herpes simplex virus infection of mother and newborn, *Pediatrics*, vol. 66, no. 4: 489–94a.

Wickett, W.H., Jr. 1976. Herpes American style, experience with Herpes simplex disease using an experimental drug. Paper presented at the 1976 meeting of the American College Health Association, Denver, Colorado.

Wickett, W.H., Jr., Bradshaw, J.L., Wilson, J., and Glasky, A.J. 1976. Clinical Effectiveness of an immuno-potentiating agent in herpes virus infections. American Society for Microbiology. (Abstract.)

Wise, T.G., Pavan, P.R., and Ennis, F.A. 1977. Herpes simplex virus vaccines, *The Journal of Infectious Diseases*, vol. 136, no. 5: 706–11.

Wohlenberg, C.R., et al. 1976. Efficacy of Phosphonoacetic acid on herpes simplex virus infection of sensory ganglia, *Infection and Immunity*, vol. 13, no. 4: 1519–21.

Wollensak, J. 1979. Herpes simplex of the eye and possibilities of its therapeutic control. *Advances in Ophthalmology*, vol. 38: 99–104. (Karger, Basel, 1979. Berlin: Free University of Berlin.)

Wolontis, S., and Jeansson, S. 1977. Correlation of Herpes simplex virus types 1 and 2 with clinical features of infection. *The Journal of Infectious Disease*, vol. 135, no. 1: 28–33.

Wright, R.A., and Judson, F.N. 1978. Relative and seasonal incidences of the sexually transmitted diseases. *British Journal of Venereal Diseases*, vol. 54: 433–40.

Young, E.J., et al. 1976. Disseminated herpevirus infection. *Journal of the American Medical Association*, vol. 235, no. 25.

zur Hausen, H. 1978. Herpes simplex virus: Benefit versus risk factors in immunization. International Symposium on Immunization, Brussels, 1978. Develop. biol. Standard. vol. 43: 373–79. (Karger, Basel, 1979.)

INDEX

Cervix, 8, 27, 34, 37, 75–76, 77, 97, 99, 109 ff., 116, 128, 138, 150, 180, 186, 187, 188, 196–201, 208–209. *See also* Cancer.

Chloroform, 149

Clitoris, 26, 30, 34, 75, 163

Codeine, 147–148

Corey, Dr. Lawrence, 157

Cortisone, 141–43

Cousins, Norman, 121

Cystitis, 100–101

Cytomegalic inclusion disease, 46, 177–180

D

Dermatomes, 82

DNA, 46, 47, 77
   virus of, 50 ff., 158, 204

Downie, Dr. Gerald, 87

Dyes, photoinactivation with, 145–146, 207

E

Eczema, 17

Estrogen, 66–67

Ether, 149

Europe, 1, 17, 55

Exercise, 130–131, 136, 137

Eye, 22, 23, 84, 104, 116, 142, 153–154, 165, 174. *See also* Keratitis

F

Fatigue, 52, 68, 69, 86, 205

Fever blisters, 1, 18–20, 22, 22, 23, 25, 27, 29 ff., 34, 37, 39–41, 52–53, 64, 67, 75, 76, 103, 116, 120, 142, 162, 164, 174, 193, 208

Fiber in diet, 135–136

Food, 67–68, 134 ff.
   diet, 52, 186–187, 210
   herpes-related, 131–133
   smoking and, 136–137

Food and Drug Administration (F.D.A.), 141, 147, 155, 170, 208

Forchet, 26, 28, 34, 75, 144

France, 169

G

Genital Herpes. *See* Herpes, genital

Germany, 157, 169

Gonorrhea, 1, 47, 55, 59, 74, 98–99, 107, 160

Gynecologists, 2, 108, 109, 138, 162, 183, 184

Gynecology, 204

H

Harris, Bert, 162

Hayden, Dr. Richard, 162

HELP, 210

Herpes (HSV)
   epidemic proportions of, 1–3, 55–59, 203, 207
   pregnancy and, 7, 37, 181–194
   infants and, 7, 8, 36–37, 39–41
   emotional aspects of, 8, 10, 11, 13–14
   simplex hominus virus, 8, 12 ff., 22, 23, 30, 47, 80, 81, 82, 85, 88, 101, 173, 209–211
   Type 1, 17, 18, 21, 22, 23, 33, 34, 35, 37, 64, 65, 71, 76, 77, 78

230

I

J

K

L

M

N

O

P

"Placebo effect," 120–121, 143, 146, 163, 164, 166 ff., 175, 179

Poliomyelitis, 80, 81, 86–90, 174, 176

Pregnancy, 7, 8, 36–37, 85, 116, 161, 181–194, 208
  natural childbirth and herpes and, 183–186
  three classes of control of herpes infection and, 192–194. *See also* Caesarian section.

Progesterone, 66–67

Prostate, 77, 117

Protein shell, 46

R

Radas, Gina, 162

Relaxation, 122–124, 186

Resistance, lowered. *See* Immune Response

RNA, 46, 159

Road Less Traveled, The, 121

S

Sabin, Dr. Albert, 86, 174, 176

Salk, Dr. Jonas, 86

Scarring, 31, 82, 164, 173

Scrotum, 29, 31, 58, 105, 115, 130, 146, 164

Settineri, Robert, 48–50

Sexual activity, 18, 27, 30, 31, 34, 68–69, 75, 76, 77, 79, 80, 98 ff., 101, 103 ff., 116 ff., 118, 163, 182, 191, 192, 195, 196, 205, 210

Shields, Dr. L. Donald, 161–162

Shingles. *See* Herpes zoster.

Smallpox vaccination, 143–145

Smoking, 62–64, 86, 136–138, 187, 204, 210

South America, 18

Sores. *See* Lesions.

Sores, canker, 20–21, 28, 65, 120, 142, 164, 204

Sores, cold. *See* Fever blisters.

Spain, 169

Stead, Elizabeth, 135

Steroids, 141–143

Stress, 17, 52, 67–69, 78, 79, 80, 120–121, 122, 150–152, 182, 184, 205, 210
  See also Herpes, emotional aspects of.

Syphilis, 1, 17, 22, 47, 55, 59, 75, 98–99, 100, 107, 141, 158
  See also Gonorrhea, Venereal disease, etc.

T

Takahashi, Dr., 174

Target cells, 93

T-helper cells, 92, 93, 94, 204

Thighs, 26, 146

T-killer cells, 92, 93, 94, 204

Tonsils, 76 ff.

Townsend, Dr. Sir Lance, 184

Trauma, 64–65, 176, 184

Treatment, local, 149–150, 156, 207
  in future, 155–171

Trigeminal nerve, 53, 65, 72, 156

Triggers, 18, 20, 21, 50, 61–70, 73, 77, 82, 89, 151, 182, 203, 205, 210
  athletic activity as, 65–66
  definition of, 19, 61
  fatigue as, 52, 69, 205
  food as, 52, 67–68, 133, 205
  menstruation as, 66–67
  nuts as, 21
  seasonal, 66, 205
  smoking as, 62–65

233

U

V

W

X

Y

Z